THE ART OF LASER ACUPUNCTURE

A Personal View

Dr. Ralph Ballard

MBBS, FAMAC

Arcadia Press

The Art of Laser Acupuncture

Published 2022

ISBN 978-0-6483772-5-2

Published by Arcadia Press
www.arcadiapress.com.au

Country of publication: Australia

Dedicated with gratitude to my mentor

Dr. Geoff Greenbaum

MBBS, FAMAC, FRACGP

Dr. Ralph Ballard

MBBS, FAMAC

Consultant Medical Acupuncturist at The Northern Hospital, Epping, Victoria, Australia 2007 – 2014

Co-Ordinator of the medical acupuncture unit in the Post Graduate Diploma of Integrative Medicine, Swinburne University. Melbourne 2001 - 2005

Assistant Medical Acupuncturist at PANCH (Preston And Northcote Community Hospital) and The Northern Hospital, Epping 1992 - 2000

Teacher for the Australian Medical Acupuncture College from 1991

Fellow of the Australian Medical Acupuncture College

ACKNOWLEDGEMENTS

My Teachers

Dr. Geoff Greenbaum

Prof. Dr. Sir Anton Jayasuriya

My Colleagues

Dr. Tim Begbie

Dr. Angela Catanzariti

Dr. Roberta Chow

Dr. Ewald Einoder

Dr. Paul Ghaie

Dr. Natasha Kustura

Dr. Ian Relf

Dr. Danny Traum

Dr. Katrina Watson

And the pioneering work of

Prof. Johannes Bischko

Dr. Felix Mann

Dr. Ian Schneideman

Contents

ABOUT THE AUTHOR

Dr. Ralph Ballard

MBBS, FAMAC

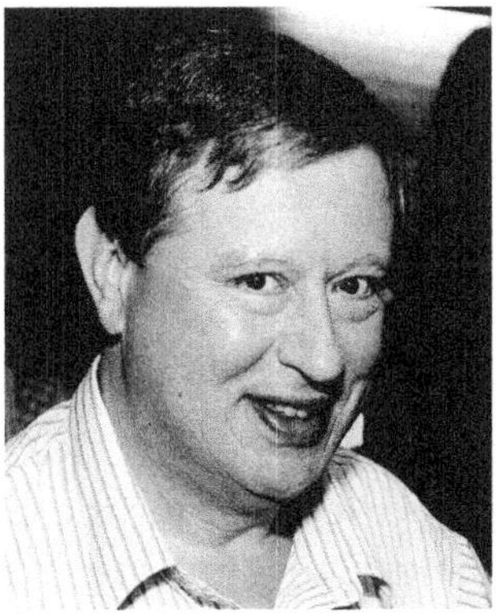

Ralph graduated in medicine from the University of Melbourne in 1982.

He then spent four years working in hospitals, and in 1987 completed training in general practice with the Family Medicine Program.

There followed a period in general practice, and then from 1990 a move into wholistic medical practice at the Whole Health Clinic, Fairfield. During this time Ralph developed an interest in a range of healing modalities and studied formally in counselling, hypnotherapy, meditation, yoga, spinal manipulation, nutritional medicine, homoeopathy, qigong, reiki, and acupuncture.

Acupuncture training began with medical acupuncture courses run by Dr. Geoff Greenbaum and Dr. Anton Jayasuriya from 1986 to 1989.

Ralph has been utilising acupuncture in his private medical practice since 1987 – some 35 years of clinical experience in medical acupuncture.

From 1988 through to 2000 Ralph assisted at the Medical Acupuncture Clinic run by Dr. Greenbaum at Preston And Northcote Community Hospital in Melbourne, then subsequently at The Northern Hospital, Epping.

Dr. Greenbaum had a particular interest in laser acupuncture and Ralph took to this keenly under Geoff's expert guidance.

In 1991 Ralph was awarded the Fellowship of the Australian Medical Acupuncture College by examination.

In 1992 he was officially appointed to the PANCH medical staff as Assistant Medical Acupuncturist.

Ralph then spent a period of time from 2001 to 2005 at Swinburne University, Melbourne as a lecturer for the Graduate School of Integrative Medicine, and as the unit co-ordinator for the medical acupuncture unit of the Post Graduate Diploma of Integrative Medicine.

From 2007 he was appointed as Consultant Medical Acupuncturist at The Northern Hospital, Epping until closure of the clinic in 2014.

Ralph has been a teacher in Geoff Greenbaum's medical acupuncture courses since 1991, including with the Monash University Graduate Certificate in Medical Acupuncture from the inception of the course until its cessation in 2013. Since that time, he has been a teacher for the Australian Medical Acupuncture College National Course, and in 2020 was appointed as an

Examiner for AMAC.

Ralph and his wife Sushie live in country Victoria on a 1-acre property near Warburton. They have two cats Marty and Moose, along with various friendly wildlife. They share a love of nature and of local community life. Ralph has played the Scottish bagpipes since early teenage years at Scotch College, Melbourne, and later with the Australian champion Hawthorn City Pipe Band. These days Ralph plays the pipes at local functions such as the Anzac Day Service, and he also plays the Scottish smallpipes and Irish whistles with local celtic musicians.

Ralph has previously contributed to a book for people with ADHD and high functioning Autism Spectrum Disorder (Asperger's Syndrome), with author Scott Alexander King. It is titled "Indigo Children and Cheeky Monkeys" and is published by Blue Angel Press.

Ralph is now keen to share his clinical experience in this book "The Art of Laser Acupuncture – A Personal View".

INTRODUCTION

This book is about a personal approach to hands-on practical acupuncture in Australia, in the context of Western scientific medicine.

This approach has evolved from teaching by various leading authorities on medical acupuncture, including Dr. Geoffrey Greenbaum (Australia), Prof. Anton Jayasuriya (Sri Lanka), Prof. Johannes Bischko (Austria), and Dr. Felix Mann (England), combined with my own clinical experience over more than 35 years.

I was fortunate to attend medical acupuncture courses run by Geoff Greenbaum and Anton Jayasuriya from 1986 onwards. I then spent some 12 years "learning at the feet of the master" as I worked at twice weekly acupuncture clinics run by Geoff Greenbaum at Preston And Northcote Community Hospital in Melbourne, then subsequently at The Northern Hospital, Epping. Geoff must have seen some ability in me because in 1992 he arranged for me to be appointed as a Clinical Assistant to the PANCH acupuncture research clinic.

There is no better way to learn acupuncture than to serve a proper apprenticeship to a recognised acupuncture teacher.

To become a master, you must first learn from a master.

So now to the current written work.

You could look at this book as a synthesis of the fundamentals of Traditional Chinese Medicine (TCM), combined with scientific research over the last 50 years, and my own personal observation and learning from the best teachers of all – the patients who come to us and trust that we will be able to assist them.

I have spent much time thinking and meditating on the issues and insights that arise in acupuncture practice, and I have hopefully come to some useful conclusions.

I will touch only briefly on the scientific research into acupuncture, including laser acupuncture, as there are already excellent textbooks, journals and websites covering these areas very well. I do not need to reinvent the wheel.

You can find relevant scientific studies about acupuncture in the References section at the end of this book.

So, I am instead writing this book in response to the requests of many doctors I have taught over the last 30 years or so. The oft repeated question comes "What is a good book on performing laser acupuncture in my practice?"

To which my reply has been "There are no good books."

And the response then follows "Well when are you going to write that book?"

So here is my reply to all these doctors – my attempt at describing a personal hands-on approach to performing laser acupuncture (and indeed all forms of acupuncture) in a Western medical setting such as Australia.

This is a book which I hope will have a place worldwide in the practice of medical acupuncture, in particular for my first love - laser acupuncture.

I trust you will find value in the thoughts contained in this book.

Dr. Ralph Ballard, November 2022

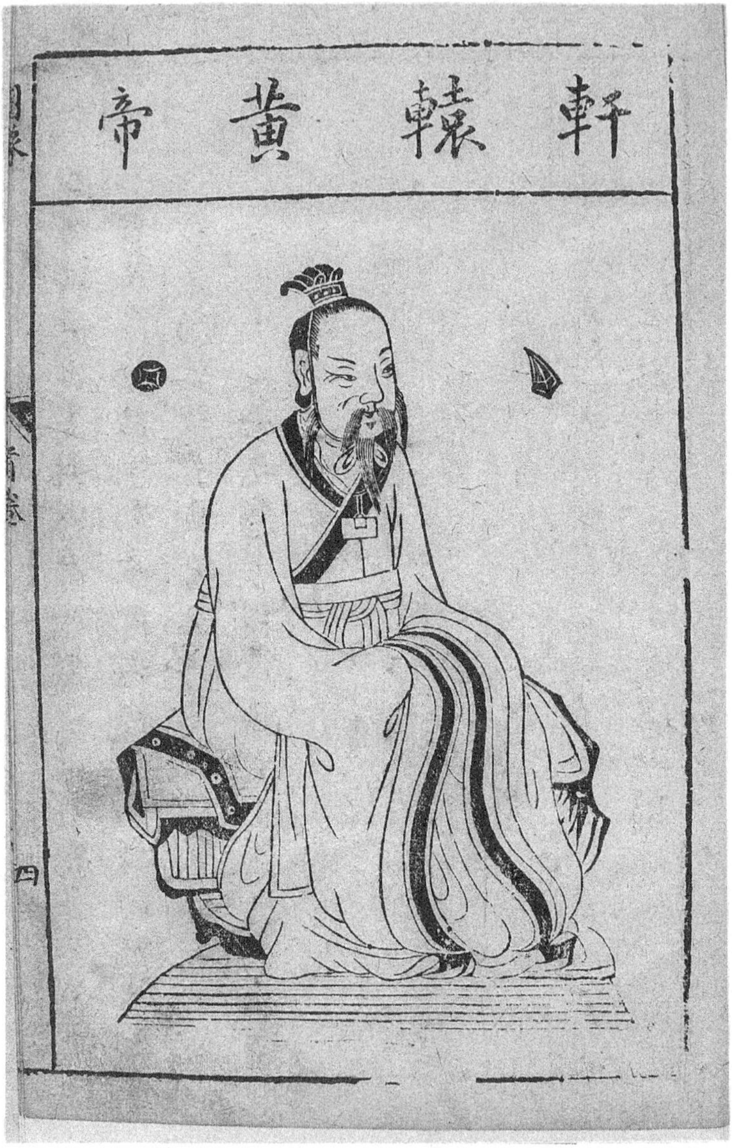

Chinese woodcut print of The Yellow Emperor

CHAPTER 1

A Brief History Of Acupuncture

Chinese traditions suggest that acupuncture is around 5,000 years old. Evidence for this comes from "Oracle Bones" housed in the Traditional Chinese Medical Museum in Beijing, China. These are animal bones inscribed with descriptions of acupuncture treatment, and have been carbon-dated to 5,000 years ago.

The first recorded Chinese texts describing acupuncture date from 200BC.

These include the Huangdi Nei Jing (The Yellow Emperor's Classic Of Internal Medicine – dated to around 200BC). This is a written collection of ancient oral teachings ascribed to the Yellow Emperor (circa 2,600BC) and his ministers, which was committed to writing in the period around 480-220BC in China.

The first part of the Huangdi Nei Jing is the Su Wen, which discusses the Taoist views of the nature of heaven, earth and the universe.

The second part is the Ling Shu. This is the first ancient text which actually describes the fundamentals of acupuncture theory and practice. It still has a very relevant and honoured place in acupuncture today.

There is also a record of acupuncture in the Shih-Chi (The Records Of The Grand Historian) written by the imperial court Grand Astrologer Sima Tan and his son Sima Qian around 100BC.

Historians Joseph Needham and Lu Gwei-djen in the 1950's and 1960's pointed out various pictographs and hieroglyphs in China dating back to 600BC showing acupuncture and moxibustion. They proposed that the earliest "acupuncture needles" were made of bone, sharpened stones, thorns or bamboo slivers.

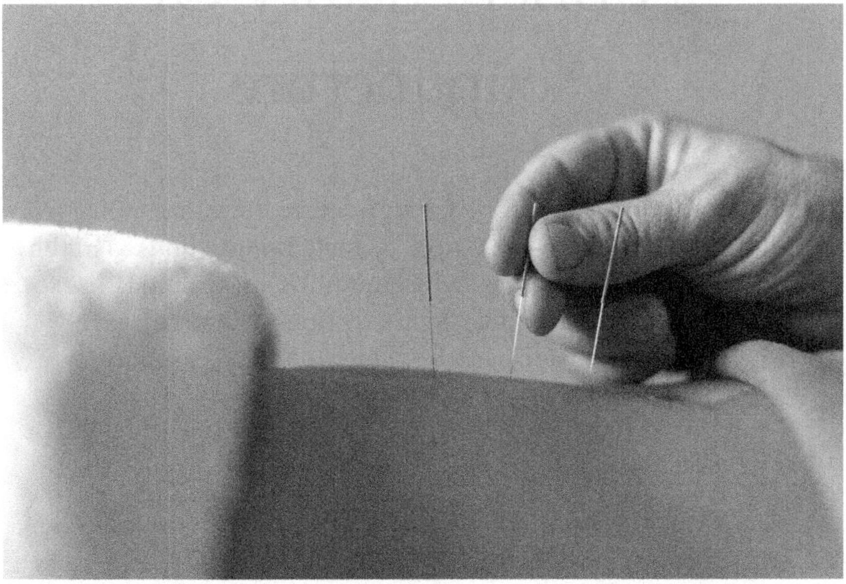

Modern day acupuncture needling (Photo courtesy of Freepik)

Sharpened stone needles known as Bian Shi have been found across China and date back to approximately 6,000 years ago in the late Neolothic Age. These sharpened stones have been particularly found in the Shandong area of eastern China. It is believed these warmed Bian Shi stones were used for acupuncture for back and neck pains. There is current scientific debate as to whether these stone needles were actually used for acupuncture, or just for simple surgery and blood-letting.

The first gold and silver needles were found in the tomb of Prince Liu Sheng dated to around 100BC.

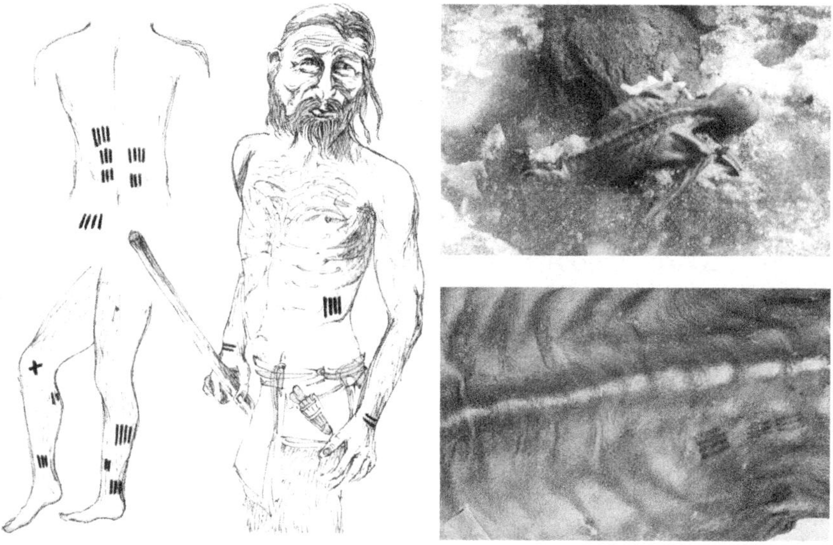

Ötzi the iceman (Photo Helmut Simon)

In another part of the world, Otzi The Iceman was found mummified in the Austrian Tyrol in 1991. He was a late Neolithic man who lived 5,300 years ago – around 3,300BC in the late Neolithic / Early Bronze Age. He was found to have puncture marks and tattoos on his body mainly grouped at recognised acupuncture points for back, knee and ankle pains, and for stomach pains. X-ray examination of his body showed degenerative arthritic changes in the lower back, knees and ankles. He was also found to have intestinal parasites which could have caused much abdominal pain. It was thought these puncture marks were made by stone needles, and so may be the earliest evidence for acupuncture – and this was in the Austrian Alps.

We have a correlation between observed maladies in the body of Otzi with the puncture marks and tattoos on his skin at known acupuncture points. Very interesting.

Did the basics of acupuncture arise in Neolithic Europe and then spread to China where it was further developed and refined? Or did it arise independently in several parts of the world? And when did it arise? Perhaps in the late Neolithic Age?

Perhaps the basics of acupuncture were in fact known extensively throughout the ancient world – whether consciously or intuitively.

Big questions.

Moving forward in time, we see that the Venetian merchant and explorer Marco Polo first brought acupuncture to Europe in 1295. It was popular in the West for a hundred years or so, but then died out.

Acupuncture was rediscovered by the Western world when President Nixon visited China in 1972. During this trip a journalist from the Washington Post accompanying the president, unexpectedly developed acute appendicitis while in China. This was too good an opportunity for the Chinese government – they organised for the appendicectomy to be performed under acupuncture anaesthesia, without pharmaceutical analgesia. All went very well and so the happy journalist wrote a front-page piece for the Washington Post.

This story "went viral" and stimulated a lot of interest throughout the Western world, including with various scientific bodies. Subsequently much university-based research was carried out into acupuncture, and this research continues to the present day.

The first question asked was "is this all fakery, or placebo?". Eventually some solid studies started to come through demonstrating a real physical effect to acupuncture beyond placebo. Since then, studies have focussed on the effects of acupuncture in various conditions, and also into exploring the mechanisms of how acupuncture works. The most powerful evidence so far is the 2012 meta-analysis by Andrew Vickers et al of some 18,000 patients which demonstrated conclusively that acupuncture is very effective for pain relief in neck and back pain, osteoarthritis, chronic headache, and shoulder pain, when compared to placebo and so-called "sham acupuncture". Subsequent review meta-analysis in 2017 showed that these benefits persist in 85% of patients.

Dr. Geoff Greenbaum was of the opinion that the ancient Chinese were excellent observers, and that they carried out their studies over an extended period of time (many hundreds of years). They used the classic scientific method of observation and testing of hypotheses over time, and made some important observations.

Firstly, it was observed that there are special reactive points on the body surface at consistent locations.

When stimulated appropriately these points produce specific reproducible effects locally, and sometimes distally in other parts of the body.

Certain very sensitive people (who we would today call Strong Responders) would sometimes experience lines of "propagated sensation" when these points were stimulated.

These lines of propagated sensation, especially when averaged out over a number of such people, would often follow specific reproducible paths on the body – this may be the basis of the Acupuncture Meridians.

You might like to read the story below about "The Prince With Migraine" to illustrate this point.

Over time Taoist then Confucianist scholars added various theories to this solid body of observed data.

As you might imagine, these academics would build on the theories that had gone before, and often tried to out-do their colleagues with all sorts of elaborations on the original data. Sometimes these theories were useful, but too often they became rather fanciful and out-of-touch with the reality of the observed data, producing confusion and distortion of the ideas. Much as happens with today's academic communities.

Acupuncture then developed over the centuries into hundreds of different approaches passed down through specific families, who often jealously guarded their "secrets".

Ultimately in the 1960's Chairman Mao, as part of the Cultural Revolution in China, ordered that all these approaches be synthesized into one grand, simple, easy-to-teach method to be given to his "barefoot doctors" so they could take this medicine out into all the villages – to give the people a cost-effective and culturally based system of national healthcare.

This became "Traditional Chinese Medicine" - TCM.

This TCM is in fact a very modern synthesis and simplification of all the ancient traditions.

The view of Traditional Chinese Medicine is that illness is due to imbalance of flow of the body's vital energy (Qi) in the organs and through the channels of the body (acupuncture meridians).

Pain is thought to be due to a build-up of stagnant Qi behind a blockage or "log-jam" in the meridian.

The acupoints are special responsive points on the meridian which can unblock or change the flow of Qi energy in that channel.

There is an excellent paper commenting on this history of TCM in "Qi, Acupuncture, and the Fascia: A Reconsideration of the Fundamental Principles of Acupuncture" by Steven and Donna Finando.

As part of the simplification process in the 1960's many interesting and "unconventional" components were removed. For example, all spiritual aspects were excluded – such as dealing with demons and possession (real, imagined or metaphorical) with such things as "Ghost Points". The reintroduction of these concepts in recent years has been very useful in using acupuncture for psychological effects as an adjunct to formal psychotherapy.

The ancient texts are still available, and some of the old wisdom is becoming available again – all useful material, subject to the provisos above about academic embellishment over time.

So, you could say that useful as the teachings of Traditional Chinese Medicine may be, it is wise not to be over-constrained by them. They are just one part of the whole story – there is much beyond the traditional teachings. Use them as a guideline when you get started with acupuncture, then explore beyond.

Observe carefully, think for yourself, build on the teachings that have been passed on to you, and draw on all the skills and wisdom you have acquired in your individual practice as a doctor/healer. Test everything against your own yardstick of clinical practice and wisdom from personal experience. And of course, take note of solid scientific research.

Then when all this is combined together, you get somewhere that is really useful. And you become much more effective as an acupuncturist.

Acupuncture continues to evolve and new discoveries are still being made.

For example, in recent years there have been fascinating developments with scalp acupuncture, new acupuncture points to treat addiction (such as the "Tim-Mee" point for tobacco smoking addiction), and the use of "Periosteal Points" from the work of Dr. Felix Mann.

And even more recently the burgeoning science of understanding the electro-chemical mechanisms of acupuncture and the functions of fascia throughout the body, are revolutionising our understandings of acupuncture. In particular, we have the possibility that transmission of signals along fascial planes may explain at least some aspects of the "classical acupuncture meridians".

The Story of "The Prince With Migraine"

There is an old story explaining the origins of acupuncture. It is probably apocryphal. I certainly hope so. You will see why when you read on.

The story goes that there was a prince in ancient China who was a bold warrior and very brave. However, he was afflicted by frequent nasty headaches (migraines in our language).

He sought the help of all the healers he could find. Practitioners from China, from India, even from Tibet.

But no one could help him.

So eventually he had to give up the search for a cure.

But he was a bold warrior and continued to fight in battle.

Then one day, when he least expected it, he was struck in the foot by an arrow. In the forefoot right between the first and second toes.

And amazingly all the headaches disappeared and never came back!

Those of you in the know will have already guessed it. This was the point we know as Taichong – Liver 3. Well known to help migraines.

Anyhow the story goes on.

From then on, prisoners of war were interviewed as to what illnesses they had. They were then lined up and arrows were randomly shot at them.

Those that survived (ugh!) were then followed up as to whether their illnesses went away, and the corresponding body points were recorded.

Over time a body of information was built up.

And so we have the origins of acupuncture.

A bit of a gruesome story, but I am sure you get the point! (Pun intended).

CHAPTER 2

The Development Of Laser Acupuncture

A History Of Light Therapy

Our Sun is the source of all life on this planet. It is literally and esoterically "The Giver Of Light" – both physically and spiritually.

Light Therapy uses this fundamental axis of life for restoring health and balance to the organism.

For millenia, many cultures have worshiped the sun as the giver of life. For example, in ancient Egypt we had the sun gods Atum and Ra, in bronze age Mesopotamia there was the sun god Shamash, in ancient Greece there were Helios and Apollo, Rome had Sol, the Incas in South America had Inti, and in ancient India, Surya was the solar deity.

Going back to the Greek physician Hippocrates in the 4th century BC, sunlight was seen as a crucial part of "hygiene" – the path to recovery. Hygeia was the Greek goddess of healing.

Hippocrates, often seen as the father of Western medicine, aimed to support the natural healing capacity of the human organism. These fundamental practices for healing included rest, healthy diet, good quality drinking water, regular bathing, and sunlight exposure.

Sunbathing and sun-gazing have been popular for many centuries worldwide as practices to heal the body and the mind.

Florence Nightingale, the great innovator in nursing care in the 1800's, declared that in her experience direct exposure to sunlight was a great aid in the healing process.

Recent 20th century work has shown that specific frequencies of light have particular effects on the human body.

An important example of this is that red light has been shown to boost cell metabolism and cell function, through the interaction of red and infra-red light with the cell's mitochondria. Here in the mitochondria red/infra-red light activates the enzyme Cytochrome C Oxidase, to produce nitrous oxide, reactive oxygen species (ROS), and ATP - the major energy source for the cell.

This work led to the development of light therapy with lasers.

LASER = Light Amplification by
Stimulated Emission of Radiation.

A laser is a beam of light produced with specific properties:

- **Monochromicity** - single wavelength (light of one colour only)
- **Coherence** (all the peaks and troughs of the waves of light are synchronised)
- **Collimation** (parallel pencil-thin beam of light)

Albert Einstein developed the theoretical basis of lasers, and published this work in 1917.

Then in the 1950's the Maser was developed, as micro-wave

amplification using the same principles as lasers.

Subsequently in 1960 the first ruby laser was developed in the USA by both Gordon Gould and by a group at Bell Laboratories led by Charles Townes and Arthur Schawlow.

Then in 1961 the 632.8nm low power red light HeNe gas laser was developed.

In 1962 the first solid state laser diodes were developed.

In 1967 Andre Mester at Semmelweis University in Budapest, Hungary, used low power red light from the HeNe laser on mice and found it promoted regrowth of hair and also wound healing. He then applied this light to humans and found it could help with healing chronic skin ulcers.

Since then lasers of various intensities have been developed.

The use of high-power laser for destructive cutting effects in surgery and industry is well known.

We also have a range of low powered lasers used in such things as CD players, bar code readers at supermarket checkouts, and as pointers in lecture theatres.

And we have the use of low power lasers for therapeutic effects on the human body. This area of medicine is now called PhotoBioModulation Therapy (PBM or PBMT). The laser can be used to reduce inflammation and tissue oedema, for chronic joint problems, healing of wounds and nerves, treating neurological problems and relieving pain by direct application of the light. These low power lasers can also be used to "stimulate" classical acupuncture points, or to de-activate trigger points in muscles, fascia, tendons, ligaments, and periosteum.

A Short History Of Laser Acupuncture

As we have seen, lasers were developed in the 1960's.

Subsequently in the mid-1970's low power HeNe lasers were applied to acupuncture by Prof. Johannes Bischko and his team at the Ludwig Boltzmann Institute For Acupuncture at the University of Vienna, Austria.

This has developed into the field of Low Level Laser Therapy (LLLT) – also known as Cold Laser Therapy, and now as PhotoBioModulation Therapy (PBM or PBMT).

Prof. Bischko was using laser doses in the order of 0.03 Joules per acupuncture point, and was getting good therapeutic effects, comparable to the results of needle acupuncture.

Subsequently Dr. Geoff Greenbaum began using Bischko's HeNe 632.8nm red light lasers and successfully introduced them to the medical acupuncture research clinic at Preston And Northcote Hospital (PANCH) in Melbourne, Australia. This clinic had originally been set up by the head of anaesthetics at the hospital, Dr. John Woodley in 1973, after he went to Hong Kong to train in the newly "discovered" modality of acupuncture. After Dr. Woodley retired, Dr. Geoff Greenbaum, who had also trained in Hong Kong with the same acupuncturist cardio-thoracic surgeon as Dr. Woodley, took over the clinic.

The work of Bischko was later confirmed by a long-term clinical study at PANCH in Melbourne, Australia. It was conducted by Dr. Geoff Greenbaum and I took part in this. This study looked at 1,000 consecutive patients presenting randomly to the acupuncture clinic at PANCH from 1985 to 2000, and assessed the results of both needle acupuncture and of Bischko's laser acupuncture. The conclusion was that both needle and laser acupuncture were effective modalities for performing acupuncture, and that benefits of each tend to persist long-term.

Since that time there has been a lot of varying data and divergent opinions about laser acupuncture – including what are the best wavelengths to use, the best laser dosages per acupuncture point, how deep does the laser penetrate, what conditions can it be effectively used for, and even does it work at all.

There is a significant difference between Laser Acupuncture and LLLT (PBMT), including in target effects and dosages applied. More on this later.

There is much still to clarify.

Suffice it to say, I am fully convinced that low level red light laser acupuncture, as per the Bischko method used at PANCH hospital, works very well for acupuncture. Since that time, I personally have seen nothing that is more effective than the Bischko / PANCH laser acupuncture method with the 1.5mW 632.8nm HeNe red light laser. This Bischko-style laser acupuncture can be used for virtually all the conditions that needles are effective for.

I will concede that acupuncture anaesthesia for surgery and for childbirth is best done with needle-based electro-acupuncture, and that sometimes needles have a quicker onset of action in acute pain (but not always).

A Strong Responder will get fast results whatever modality is used for acupuncture. More on Strong Responders in a later chapter.

My old Bischko-style Silberbauer 1.5mW laser wore out years ago and is no longer commercially available. So I use the next best thing – a Silberbauer 8mW 658nm red light CL Mini-Lase with a power reducing tip, delivering 0.06 Joules per acupuncture point. A very suitable compact laser for acupuncture, providing excellent therapeutic results in my hands.

There is some good recent scientific work indicating that in general laser doses of around 0.5 Joules per point delivered by a continuous red-light laser are perhaps optimal in most situations.

However, I am by nature a minimalist, and I prefer the lowest dose possible. I find this works really well with my patients. Given that I am a sensitive Strong Responder myself, I do of course draw patients to me who are typically also sensitive Strong Responders. And I expect my patients to respond very well to my minimalist treatment. Just as Dr. Felix Mann found in his clinical work. More on Dr. Mann later.

"Birds of a feather flock together."

This is a well-known aphorism that applies very well in acupuncture practice. You will tend to draw to you patients who match your expectations and your own innate responsiveness.

But I digress.

CHAPTER 3

Scientific Evidence for Qi

Ancient Concepts

3,000 BC – Concept of ***Prana***, universal life force, in India.

This understanding was applied in the practice of yoga and meditation.

1,000 BC – Qigong Masters in China used meditation to build their life force ***Qi*** to balance and invigorate health.

Movement disciplines (Tai Chi, Qigong, etc) and martial arts, as well as acupuncture, were developed to work with this energy.

500 BC – Pythagoras taught about the universal energy throughout nature which could be used for healing.

In the early centuries AD, Neo-Platonic & Jewish Kabbalah scholars talked about the ***Astral Light*** around people.

Later Christian teachers spoke of the ***Halo*** around great spiritual people – shown in Christian paintings.

Renaissance Concepts

1500's - Paracelsus (Swiss-German physician, and founder of toxicology) developed the concept of Yliaster – an energy or prime substance which humans have, comprised of both matter and a vital force.

Early 1600's – Jan Baptist van Helmont (Flemish chemist and physician) talked about a universal spiritual fluid pervading all living beings.

Enlightenment Concepts

Early 1800's – Dr. Franz Mesmer in Germany developed hypnosis on the basis that a fluid electromagnetic field existed around the human body. This field naturally transferred between all animate beings and inanimate objects – animal magnetism. Mesmer believed he could influence people through manipulating this field.

Late 1880's – The French scholars Emile Boirac and Ambroise-Augsuste Liebeault said that each person has an energy which reacts with other people either harmoniously or negatively. They conducted experiments on Animal Magnetism and the phenomena of hypnosis.

The Human Energy Field

The Human Energy Field (HEF) is the name often used in modern research, for the Qi of the human body.

History of Research into the HEF

Mid 1800's – Count Wilhelm von Reichenbach did experimental work showing an electromagnetic field around the human body - called the Odic Field.

This field was similar to the electromagnetic fields described by James Maxwell in the 1880's.

Reichenbach showed that with this Odic Field, like attracts like.

Electro-positive Elements produce feelings of warmth and distress.

Electro-negative Elements produced sensations of coolness and peace.

Odic force could be conducted through a wire at 13 feet per second.

1911 – Dr. Walter Kilner MD (St. Thomas Hospital, London) reported an energy field or aura around the human body when viewed through glass stained with dicyanin dye.

This aura varied according to race, sex, level of health, and various emotional states.

Changes in the visualised aura could be used to diagnose various illnesses.

Reference book - "The Human Aura" by Dr. Walter Kilner. 1965. New York.

Dr. Wilhelm Reich – psychiatrist/psychoanalyst following on from Dr. Sigmund Freud.

In the 1930's to 1950's Reich studied the universal energy field – a cosmic energy he called Orgone Energy.

In the 1940's he developed "Orgone Accumulators" to enhance this life force in people.

This Accumulator was an insulated Faraday Cage with walls of alternating plywood, rock wool and sheet iron.

In 1942 published his book "The Discovery of the Orgone"

Harold Saxon Burr (Professor of Anatomy at Yale University School of Medicine) during the 1930's – 1960's experimented with an electromagnetic field he found permeating all living tissue.

Burr used a voltmeter to detect the electrical potential of the human body in 1936.

He subsequently found this bio-electrical field in all living things, and measured consistent changes with cell replication.

He considered that this electrical field determined cell differentiation, and the form of all living organisms.

1940's – 1960's – Semyon Kirlian (electrical engineer in Russia) and his wife Valentina Kirlian, observed high energy electrical discharges between high frequency electrical equipment and human beings.

They placed photographic plates in the path of the electrical discharge and produced photos of "the aura" of plants as well as people.

They famously produced photos showing a residual image of a complete leaf after the leaf had been cut in half – the so-called "phantom leaf effect".

Dr. George De La Warr and Dr. Ruth Brown in England researched radiation emitted from living tissues and built a "Radionic machine" to measure this. They were able to accurately diagnose various disease states from hair samples.

Dr. De La Warr published his work in the books "Biomagnetism" 1965 and "Using Sound Waves to Probe Matter" 1967.

Dr. Robert Becker (orthopaedic surgeon) at Upstate Medical School (USA) mapped an electrical energy field corresponding to the form of the human body and CNS (central nervous system).

In 1962 he called this electrical field "the direct current control system". All cells and animals were found to have a direct current of electric charge which was measurable on the body surface.

Becker's research showed that this electrical field changed shape and strength according to the individual's physiological and psychological state, and that particles the size of electrons moved through the field.

Reference: The Body Electric. Dr. Robert Becker. 1985.

Dr. Zheng Ronliang of Lanzhou University, China, measured Qi radiated from the human body with a biological detector made from a leaf vein connected to a photo quantum device.

He studied Qi radiating from a Qigong Master, and the energy field emanating from a clairvoyant.

Dr. Ronliang found that the Qigong Master sometimes radiated Qi with a very low frequency carrier wave, and at other times radiated Qi as a 60 micron sized particle with a velocity of 20-50 cm/sec.

The clairvoyant's energy emissions were very different to this.

Reference: Scientific Research of Qigong. Dr. Zhen Ronliang.

Scientists at the Bioinformation Institute of the Popov Academy, Russia, announced the discovery that all living organisms emit energy in the wavelength range of 300 – 2000 nanometers.

They called this energy Bioplasma.

This bio-field was found to be stronger in people who were able to transfer their bio-energy.

Scientists at the Medical Sciences Academy in Moscow later confirmed these findings.

Dr. Victor Inyushin at Kazakh University, Russia, published works in the 1960's on his research into Bioplasma energy as a fifth state of matter (the standard 4 states are solids, liquids, gases, and plasma).

He showed that Bioplasma particles are constantly renewed by chemical cellular processes, and these Bioplasma particles are in constant motion.

In disease an imbalance is seen between positive and negative Bioplasma particles.

Dr. William Tiller (physicist and Professor in Materials Science and Engineering at Stanford University 1964 - 1992) predicted in 1987 that bio-electricity would be the next phase of medical technology to assess and treat the human mind and body.

He based this prediction on the understanding that all vital systems operate electrically as well as chemically.

Cellular and intra-cellular structures, cell membranes, connective tissue, tendons, ligaments, and fascia all have an electrical potential, and so create and conduct electrical currents.

In the 1970's and 1980's Dr. Valerie Hunt at UCLA (USA) found consistent correlation between "aura colours" seen by 8 clairvoyants, with specific variations from EMG readings with electrodes placed over the chakra locations.

Specific EMG patterns correlated with specific aura colours.

Her work showed that the human energy field, especially in healers, showed patterns of high coherence when analysed by chaos computer programs.

Reference: A Study of Structural Neuromuscular, Energy Field and Emotional Approaches, Dr. Valerie Hunt and Wayne Massey, UCLA, 1977.

Prof. Rupert Sheldrake (biochemist and cell biologist at Cambridge University 1967 – 1973) has researched Morphic Resonance. Morphic Resonance suggests that "memory is inherent in nature" and "natural systems, such as termite colonies, or pigeons, or orchid plants, or insulin molecules, inherit a collective memory from all previous things of their kind". Prof. Sheldrake proposed that it is also responsible for "telepathy-type interconnections between organisms". He developed the concept of Morphogenetic Fields – organisational control fields of group consciousness.

In Germany Dr. Reinhard Voll in the 1950's developed a form of electro-acupuncture (EAV) to measure electrical skin resistance at certain acupuncture points, and the changes in this electrical skin resistance in various disease states.

Helmut Schimmel developed this technique further in the 1970's as Vega Testing. This approach claims to diagnose disease states and various functional disturbances in the body such as allergies.

Dr. Franz Morell subsequently developed Mora Therapy as a more sophisticated diagnostic and treatment system.

Hiyoshi Motoyama PhD (Japan) in the 1970's measured light emitted from long-term yoga practitioners.

This low-level photon emission was recorded on movie cameras in a darkroom.

His further research showed that:

A healer's energy dipped while giving energy to another, then rose again afterwards.

In particular, the heart energy of a healer increased after treating a patient.

Reference: The Functional Relationship Between Yoga Asanas and Acupuncture Meridians. Hiyoshi Motoyama. 1979.

August 2005 – Nakamura & Hiramatsu (Japan) reported the measurable emission of photons from the human hand, especially the fingernails.

This light emission varies in different disease states and may become a useful diagnostic tool.

Professor Fritz-Albert Popp, an expert on biologically related photons at the International Institute of Biophysics in Germany, has done parallel work which supports these findings.

Reference - J Photochem Photobiol B. 2005 Aug 1;80(2):156-60. Ultra-weak photon emission from human hand: influence of temperature and oxygen concentration on emission. Nakamura K, Hiramatsu M. http://www.ncbi.nlm.nih.gov/pubmed/15935689

Building Qi

Qigong is the practice of working with and building your own Qi.

The regular practice of Qigong is believed to enhance health, treat illness, and produce a long happy life.

Time spent in nature, in meditation, and in quiet retreat can also build Qi.

Correct diet and certain herbs can assist with building Qi too.

Qigong Masters can project their Qi with powerful effects.

Medical Qigong

Advanced Qigong practitioners can project their Qi for healing.

This can be used to enhance the effect of acupuncture treatment.

This is akin to Dr. Geoff Greenbaum's quote about the therapeutic benefit of "the doctor's healing hands".

Good doctors/healers can help their patients just by being with them, especially when touching them.

A video of Qigong practitioners shrinking a bladder tumour at a Chinese hospital can be seen at https://youtu.be/31rf74-DQfA

Summary of Qi

Over the last 150 years various scientific researchers have provided evidence that the human body possesses a subtle invisible energy field.

This equates to evidence for the human body's Qi.

This human energy field can interact with others and have either a harmonising or disturbing effect.

This field can project Qi or energy to others for healing.

General Reference: "Vibrational Medicine" by Dr. Richard Gerber MD. Third Edition 2001. Bear & Company. Rochester, Vermont.

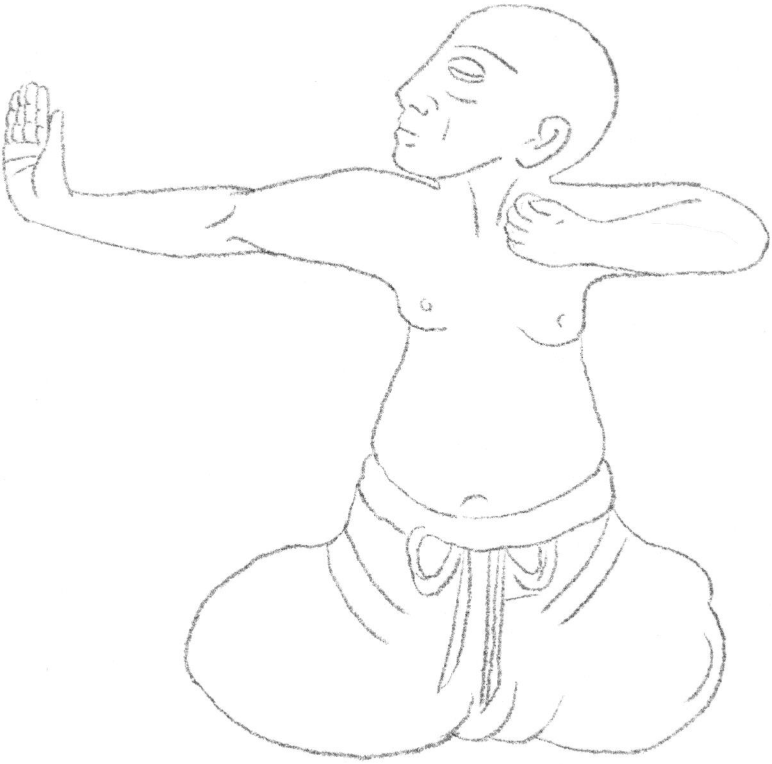

Qigong - projecting Qi

CHAPTER 4

What Is An Acupuncture Point

In simple terms, an acupuncture point is a sensitive point on the body surface.

This specific sensitivity to stimulus means that a range of effects can be produced that do not occur when stimulating other parts of the body.

As examples of the particular sensitivity of acupuncture points, they are often sensitive to pressure and can be detected by a change in electrical skin conductivity when measured by a galvanometer.

Stimulation of this reactive acupuncture point can produce specific reproducible effects on the body, both locally and distally (in other parts of the body). This response is usually felt as pain relief, but other effects may also occur.

The acupuncture point is typically in the region of pain and is generally close to a significant nerve branch.

This location is often deep in the muscle belly or at the end of a muscle where it attaches to a bone (the teno-periosteal junction).

Dr. Peter Dorsher from the Mayo Clinic Florida in the USA has recently done important work on the physical make-up of acupuncture points and has confirmed they consist of four components:

1. A collection of A-delta and C nerve fibres (specialised sensory nerve endings)

2. A collection of Mast Cells (white cells which release histamine to cause inflammation in response to external invaders such as allergens or parasites)

3. A collection of Fibroblasts (cells which produce connective tissue as a structural framework in the body)

4. All of these components are based in a neuro-vascular bundle (a collection of nerves and blood vessels wound together)

In other words, an acupuncture point is basically a 1-2mm collection of A-delta and C fibres surrounded by mast cells and fibroblasts, penetrating a pore in the fascia/muscle/bone, and adjacent to a local neuro-vascular bundle. This was first demonstrated in 1979 by Senelar and has been confirmed by further studies since then.

See Chapter 3 "Myofascial Pain" by Dr Peter Dorsher in "Pain – The person, the science, the clinical interface" edited by Patricia Armati and Roberta Chow. IP Communications. Melbourne. 2015.

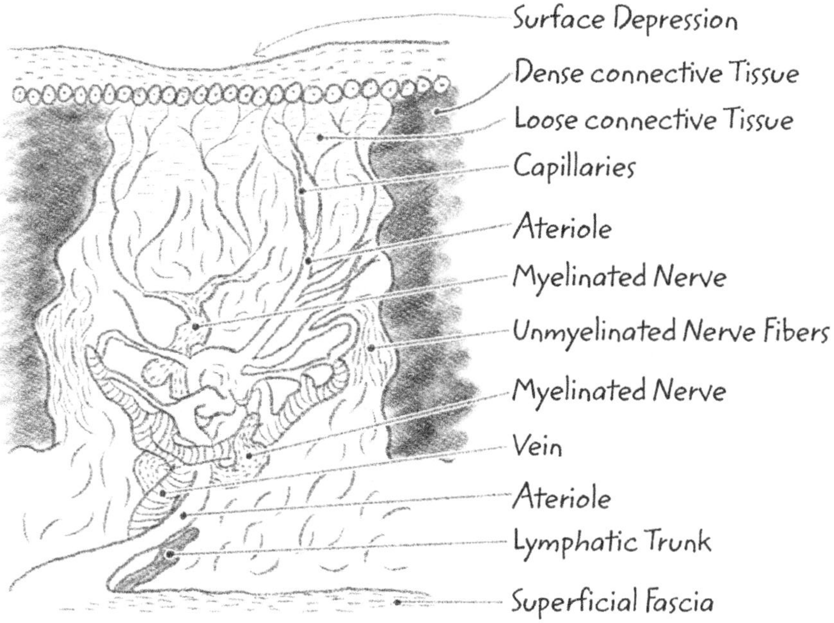

Typical histological structure of an acupuncture point.

In addition, Wei Zhou has recently demonstrated that at least some of the major acupuncture points overlie major nerve bundles.

> See "Zhou W, Benharash P. Effects and mechanisms of acupuncture based on the principle of meridians. J Acupunct Meridian Stud. 2014 Aug;7(4):190-3. doi: 10.1016/j.jams.2014.02.007."

Another view of acupuncture points has been demonstrated by Kirlian photography where energy flares can be seen at acupuncture points when photographed under a high-voltage high-frequency electrical field in a darkened room.

An acupuncture point can be treated at 3 main levels:

1. Deep in the body tissues

This is typically based on stimulating De Qi – the "acupuncture Qi sensation" felt when the needling is effective. In Western scientific terms, this is stimulating specific nerve endings. Is this effect also based on stimulating specific fascial planes? On occasion this stimulation may go deep into the periosteum covering the surface of the bone, but more commonly may be into the motor end plate in the middle of the muscle belly, or into the junction between tendons and periosteum (the teno-periosteal junction). This is the typical form of acupuncture developed in China.

2. Superficial

This involves brief penetration of the uppermost layers of the skin (as in Japanese acupuncture), or simply stimulating the nerve fibrils just under the skin surface which project from the nerve endings (C and A-delta fibres) with no penetration of the actual body surface (laser acupuncture).

3. Above the skin

This involves treating the energy flare from the acupoint (as seen on Kirlian photography and its variants) and is based on projecting Qi or use of "healing hands".

This issue of depth of penetration and type of stimulation needs much more research.

CHAPTER 5

What Are The Meridians

The traditional view of the meridians is that they are lines of Qi (energy) flow in the tissues of the body, which control how the body and the mind work.

If there is a blockage in Qi flow in a meridian, or an excess / deficient Qi state in a given meridian, then disturbance in function of the mind / body can manifest. If this becomes severe enough over a prolonged period of time, then actual physical disease can manifest.

In this view acupuncture works by correcting Qi flow through the meridians.

From the Western scientific view, it has been hard to establish what the meridians actually are.

It has been observed for a number of years that propagated sensation can occur when acupuncture points are stimulated (Dr. Felix Mann) and that often these patterns of referred pain do follow the path of specific meridians.

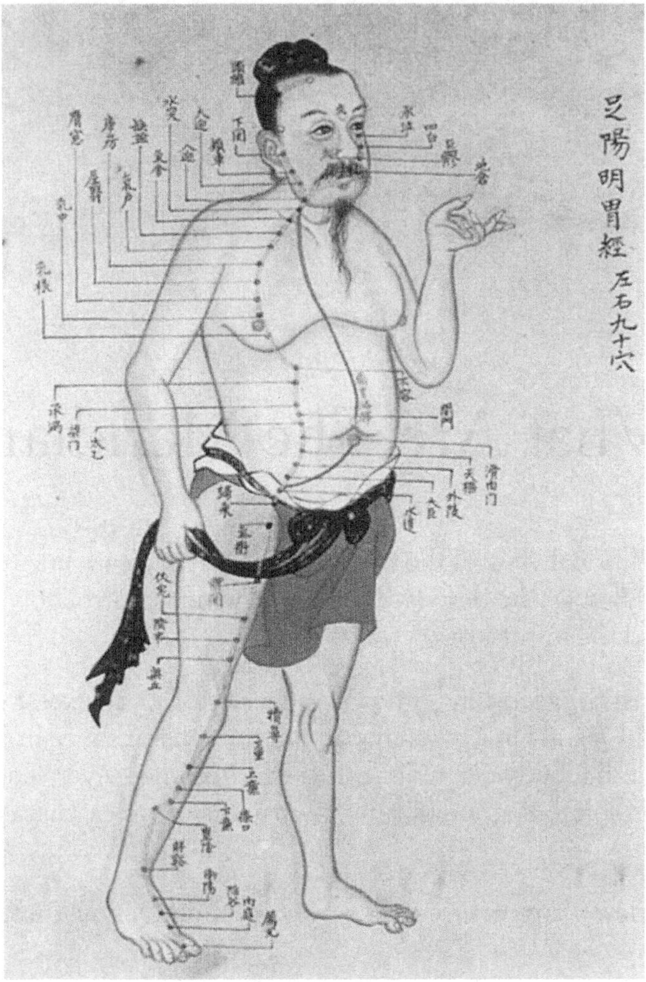

Stomach meridian

Recent scientific work by Dr. Peter Dorsher has validated this observation.

> See "Dorsher PT. Myofascial referred-pain data provide physiologic evidence of acupuncture meridians. J Pain. 2009 Jul; 10(7):723-31."

In addition, Peter Dorsher has suggested that acupuncture meridians correspond to the major nerve trunks, and that the meridians may indeed be the nerves themselves.

See "Dorsher PT, Chiang P. Neuroembryology of the Acupuncture Principal Meridians: Part 3. The Head and Neck. Med Acupunct. 2018 Apr 1; 30 (2):80-88."

Another view put forth by Steven Finando and others suggests that lines of electrical transmission along the planes of fascia separating muscles and around organs, may provide a pathway for at least some of the acupuncture meridians.

See "Qi, Acupuncture, and the Fascia: A Reconsideration of the Fundamental Principles of Acupuncture" by Steven Finando, PhD, LAc, and Donna Finando, MS, LAc, LMT. The Journal Of Alternative And Complementary Medicine, Volume 18, Number 9, 2012, pp. 880–886."

Also see "Bianco G. Fascial neuromodulation: an emerging concept linking acupuncture, fasciology, osteopathy and neuroscience. Eur J Transl Myol. 2019 Aug 27;29(3):8331. doi: 10.4081/ejtm.2019.8331. PMID: 31579478; PMCID: PMC6767840."

In addition, in the 1960's there was work done in North Korea by Kim Bong-Han suggesting that a network of tiny vessels throughout the body provided the basis for the acupuncture meridians. This network was later called the Primo Vascular System. These microscopic vessels surround blood and lymphatic vessels as well as organs. Fluorescent tracer dye was injected into various acupuncture points and could be seen to flow to other related points on the same meridian – for example injecting the LR9 point in rats resulted in the dye being detected at the rat's LR3. Kim Bong-Han's work later fell into disregard.

See "Kim, Bong-Han. "Developmental and Comparative Biological Study of Primo Vascular System". Journal of Acupuncture and Meridian Studies. 5 (5): 248–255. doi:10.1016/j.jams.2012.07.016"

CHAPTER 6

Scientific Studies On Acupuncture

General Acupuncture Studies

Firstly, regarding acupuncture in general, there are a wealth of studies on needle acupuncture.

In summary, acupuncture has been shown to be an effective modality across a range of conditions. Its mechanisms of action have been well demonstrated, and we are continuing to discover more about how it works.

Perhaps the best scientific review demonstrating the effectiveness of acupuncture is the meta-analysis by Vickers et al in 2012. This was a review of the individual patient data of nearly 18,000 patients from 29 randomised control trials and clearly showed that acupuncture was effective for pain relief in chronic headache, neck and back pain, shoulder pain and osteoarthritis, to a high degree of significance statistically. True acupuncture was also shown to be more effective than sham acupuncture.

A brief overview of how acupuncture works is:

Scientific research has found that there are specific nerve endings (A-delta fibres) at acupuncture points (acupoints) and these can be stimulated so they send signals to the spinal cord and brain to block transmission of pain impulses.

Acupuncture also sends signals to stimulate the brain to produce certain chemicals (neuropeptides) for pain relief (endorphins), to improve sleep and relieve depression (serotonin), and to provide anti-inflammatory, anti-allergy, immune-boosting and vitality-boosting effects (cortisol).

Acupuncture also sends signals from the brain back down the spinal cord to rebalance muscle function and reduce muscle spasm. This can help in chronic pain and in recovery from stroke or head injury.

Acupuncture can stimulate the brain to rebalance function of the autonomic nervous system, which controls the function of organs, nerves, and blood vessels.

Acupuncture can also restore distorted pain perceptions in the brain (neruro-plasticity).

For more detail I refer you to the References section, especially the textbooks:

"Medical Acupuncture – A Western Scientific Approach" edited by Jacqueline Filshie and Adrian White

"An Introduction To Western Medical Acupuncture" edited by Adrian White, Mike Cummings and Jacqueline Filshie

The work of Dr. Peter Dorsher quoted online and in "Pain – The person, the science, the clinical interface" edited by Patricia Armati and Roberta Chow.

Laser Acupuncture Studies

Studies on the effectiveness of laser acupuncture

The first major study into the clinical effectiveness of laser acupuncture was published in 2002. In that year Dr. Geoff Greenbaum did a presentation at ICMART (the international body for medical acupuncture) of the results of a 15-year study of 1,000 patients who presented consecutively at the PANCH acupuncture clinic. There was no standardisation of patients, of conditions, or of points used. It was an extended Case Series looking at what acupuncture can do.

I was privileged to take part in this study as one of the treating practitioners.

Positive Evidence for Laser Acupuncture

"15 Year Prospective Trial of Acupuncture in a Hospital Out-Patient Clinic with 1058 patients". ICMART 2002 Presentation Dr. Geoff Greenbaum. PANCH, Victoria, Australia.

Statistical analysis showed that both laser (Silberbauer HeNe laser delivering 0.03 Joules per point) and needling are effective modalities for acupuncture.

Response to acupuncture treatment tended to be maintained long-term. Further clinical improvements may occur 1 to 5 years after acupuncture.

The median number of treatments for successful outcome across a number of conditions was 8 – 12 treatments.

The median trend in clinical improvement across a range of conditions - generally good improvements were seen over the first 2 to 3 sessions, then a plateau in response over the next 3 to 5 sessions, then further improvement from treatments 7 to 8 and ongoing.

"Clinical effectiveness of laser acupuncture: a systematic review" G David Baxter , Chris Bleakley, Suzanne

McDonough. J Acupunct Meridian Stud. 2008 Dec;1(2):65-82.

"Evidence was found to support the use of laser acupuncture in the treatment of myofascial pain, postoperative nausea and vomiting and for the relief of chronic tension headache.

Laser acupuncture would appear to represent an effective form of acupuncture for the management of these conditions and could be considered as a viable alternative to more traditional forms of acupuncture point stimulation."

"Laser Acupuncture: Effectiveness Depends upon Dosage" G David Baxter. Acupuncture In Medicine. Volume 27 Issue 3, September 2009.

"In the treatment of chronic low back pain .... a key point to determine the effectiveness of laser acupuncture is the dosage applied.

Dosage guidelines for laser acupuncture is confounded by the lack of a clear understanding of the mechanisms underpinning such treatment.

The use of higher treatment dosages are also supported by findings from our recent systematic review of laser acupuncture trials.

This reported that dosages in previous studies of laser acupuncture for the treatment of low back pain (n = 9 studies) varied from 0.57 J to 5 J per point for positive studies.

Thus, while the definitive dosage window for effective laser acupuncture may remain occult, it is clear that higher dosages, and probably 0.5 J per point, are indicated."

"Efficacy of low-level laser therapy in the management of neck pain: a systematic review and meta-analysis of randomised placebo or active-treatment controlled trials".

Roberta Chow, Mark Johnson, Rodrigo Lopes-Martins, Jan Bjordal. Lancet 2009 Dec 5; 374(9705):1897-908.

"Neck pain is a common and costly condition for which pharmacological management has limited evidence of efficacy and side-effects.

Low-level laser therapy (LLLT) is a relatively uncommon, non-invasive treatment for neck pain, in which non-thermal laser irradiation is applied to sites of pain.

We did a systematic review and meta-analysis of randomised controlled trials to assess the efficacy of LLLT in neck pain.

We identified 16 randomised controlled trials including a total of 820 patients.

We show that LLLT reduces pain immediately after treatment in acute neck pain and up to 22 weeks after completion of treatment in patients with chronic neck pain."

"The nuts and bolts of low-level laser (light) therapy" Hoon Chung, Tianhong Dai, Sulbha K Sharma, Ying-Ying Huang, James D Carroll, Michael R Hamblin. Ann Biomed Eng. 2012 Feb;40(2):516-33.

"Soon after the discovery of lasers in the 1960s it was realized that laser therapy had the potential to improve wound healing and reduce pain, inflammation and swelling.

In recent years the field sometimes known as photobiomodulation has broadened to include light-emitting diodes and other light sources, and the range of wavelengths used now includes many in the red and near infrared.

The term "low level laser therapy" or LLLT has become widely recognized and implies the existence of the biphasic dose response or the Arndt-Schulz curve.

This review will cover the mechanisms of action of LLLT at a cellular and at a tissular level and will summarize the various light sources and principles of dosimetry that are employed in clinical practice.

The range of diseases, injuries, and conditions that can be benefited by LLLT will be summarized with an emphasis on those that have reported randomized controlled clinical trials.

Serious life-threatening diseases such as stroke, heart attack, spinal cord injury, and traumatic brain injury may soon be amenable to LLLT therapy."

A superb review of the scientific literature on PhotoBioModulation and Low Level Laser Therapy.

"Laser acupuncture for treating musculoskeletal pain: a systematic review with meta-analysis." Dina Law, Suzanne McDonough, Chris Bleakley, George David Baxter, Steve Tumilty. Journal of Acupuncture and Meridian Studies. Volume 8, Issue 1, February 2015, Pages 2-16.

"Positive effects for both pain and functional outcomes were more consistently seen at long-term follow-up rather than immediately after treatment.

Moderate-quality evidence supports the effectiveness of laser acupuncture in managing musculoskeletal pain when applied in an appropriate treatment dosage; however, the positive effects are seen only at long-term follow-up and not immediately after the cessation of treatment."

"Shining light on the head: Photobiomodulation for brain disorders" Michael R. Hamblin BBA Clin. 2016 Dec; 6: 113–124. Elsevier.

"Photobiomodulation (PBM) describes the use of red or near-infrared light to stimulate, heal, regenerate, and protect tissue that has either been injured, is degenerating, or else is at risk of dying.

One of the organ systems of the human body that is most necessary to life, and whose optimum functioning is most worried about by humankind in general, is the brain.

The brain suffers from many different disorders that can be classified into three broad groupings: traumatic events (stroke, traumatic brain injury, and global ischemia), degenerative diseases (dementia, Alzheimer's and Parkinson's), and psychiatric disorders (depression, anxiety, post traumatic stress disorder).

There is some evidence that all these seemingly diverse conditions can be beneficially affected by applying light to the head.

There is even the possibility that PBM could be used for cognitive enhancement in normal healthy people.

In this transcranial PBM (tPBM) application, near-infrared (NIR) light is often applied to the forehead because of the better penetration (no hair, longer wavelength).

Some workers have used lasers, but recently the introduction of inexpensive light emitting diode (LED) arrays has allowed the development of light emitting helmets or "brain caps".

This review will cover the mechanisms of action of photobiomodulation to the brain, and summarize some of the key pre-clinical studies and clinical trials that have been undertaken for diverse brain disorders."

The is another superb review of the scientific literature on PhotoBioModulation and Low Level Laser Therapy, specifically as it applies to treating chronic brain injuries and diseases.

Research Studies into the Mechanisms of Action of Laser Acupuncture

Research into how Laser Acupuncture works

- Laser Acupuncture works primarily through effects on nerves.
- It can cause direct neural blockade, similar to local anaesthetic.
- It seems to inhibit both A-delta and C nociceptive nerve fibres.
- This is different to needle acupuncture which inhibits C-fibres but stimulates A-delta fibres.
- It blocks Fast Axonal Flow in the nerve fibres by disrupting ATP.
- It increases micro-circulatory changes.
- It can produce transmission of electric currents along fascia planes.
- It has effects on the body's electrical fields.
- It can induce Calcium waves, both within and outside the cell.
- It can induce Stem Cell activation.
- It can induce a collagen response to assist wound healing.
- It can alter gene expression.
- It can transmit along microtubules.

Both needle and laser acupuncture work via effects on nerves.

However, the mechanisms are different.

Needle acupuncture works primarily via an electro-chemical effect on specific nerves.

The current evidence is that laser acupuncture works via a different effect on the nervous system – it produces changes in the cyto-skeleton of the peripheral nerve axon, proceeding all the way to the dorsal horn of the spinal cord.

CHAPTER 7

Laser Types

The original lasers were Helium-Neon gas tubes through which an electric current was passed, causing the gas mixture to produce photons. Eventually this photon flux would build to a sufficient level to be emitted from the end of the laser tube as a pencil-thin beam of coherent red light.

This has been followed by a range of solid diode lasers which are more robust and compact. When stimulated by an electric current they can produce light at a specific wavelength / frequency – typically visible red or invisible near-infrared light.

Laser Classification

Class 1 Laser

Safe under all conditions of normal use.

Class 2 Laser

Class 2 lasers are safe because the blink reflex will limit the eye exposure to no more than 0.25 seconds. This only applies to visible-light lasers (400–700 nm). It is also limited to 1 mW continuous wave lasers, or more if the emission time is less than 0.25 seconds, or if the light beam is not spatially coherent.

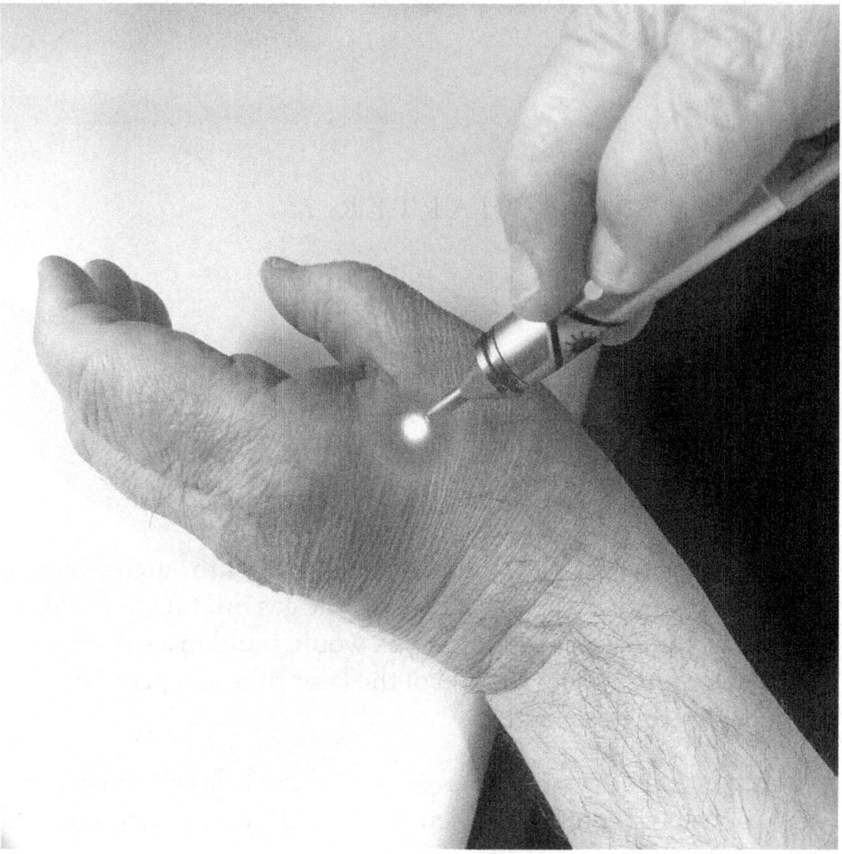

Laser Acupuncture on LI 4

Class 2M Laser

Laser beams with a large diameter or large divergence, and where the amount of light passing through the pupil does not exceed the limits for class 2.

Class 3 Laser

Potentially hazardous

Class 3R Laser

Class 3R lasers are considered safe if handled carefully, with restricted beam viewing. Visible continuous lasers limited to no more than 5mW.

Class 3B Laser

Class 3B laser is hazardous if the eye is exposed directly, but diffuse reflections such as those from paper or other matte surfaces are not harmful. Protective eyewear is typically required where direct viewing of a class 3B laser beam may occur. Class 3B lasers must be equipped with a key switch and a safety interlock.

Class 4 Laser

The highest and most dangerous class of laser, including all lasers that exceed the Class 3B parameters.

By definition, a class 4 laser can burn the skin, or cause devastating and permanent eye damage as a result of direct, diffuse or indirect beam viewing. These lasers may ignite combustible materials, and thus may represent a fire risk. These hazards may also apply to indirect or non-specular reflections of the beam, even from apparently matte surfaces — meaning that great care must be taken to control the beam path.

Class 4 lasers must be equipped with a key switch and a safety interlock. Most industrial, scientific, military, and medical lasers are in this category.

CHAPTER 8

Laser Parameters For Acupuncture

Medium:	Gas or Diode
Wavelength:	Visible Red or Infrared Invisible
Power:	mW or W (milliWatts or Watts)
Spot Size:	Continuous or Pulsed Beam. In practice most laser acupuncture currently uses a continuous laser beam. However, there is interesting laboratory research taking place into the possible benefits of pulsed laser beams.
Energy Produced:	Power (Watts) x Time (Seconds) = Joules
Energy Density:	Joules per Spot size (Joules per cm2)
Power Density:	Power per spot size (Watts per cm2)

To avoid thermal injury, use a Power Density less than 200mW per cm2.

CHAPTER 9

Laser Dosage

Low dose laser acupuncture relies on the specific properties of acupuncture points. It usually uses laser doses in the range of 0.03 to 0.5 Joules per point (although on occasion doses may go up to 1.0 Joules per point).

> As an example of laser dosage, using the formula Energy Produced: Power (Watts) x Time (Seconds) = Joules
>
> An 8mW Silberbauer Laser (wavelength 658nm) applied for 15 seconds produces a dose per point of 0.12 Joule (0.008 x 15 = 0.12).

Low Level Laser Therapy (LLLT) operates at a higher order of magnitude and acts directly on body tissues to have analgesic, anti-inflammatory and tissue healing effects. LLLT typically uses laser doses in the range of 1 to 10 Joules per point, and often employs infra-red higher power lasers.

The parameters of Energy Density and Power Density are generally more important for LLLT, wound healing and tendinopathies, but not for laser acupuncture.

CHAPTER 10

Laser Safety

Scientific research has shown that low power red light and infra-red lasers (power range 1 to 100mW, wavelength 630 to 950nm, application time 1 to 60 seconds) used in acupuncture do not cause any tissue damage, either in the short or long term. They do not cause burns and are safe for the body. Research to confirm the safety and effectiveness of these acupuncture lasers has been carried out originally at the University Of Vienna, and by many scientific institutions since then.

Laser acupuncture should NOT be applied:

- Directly into the open eye
- Over cancer tissue
- Over openings in the skull
- To the belly of a pregnant woman
- Over electronic implants – pacemakers etc.
- On the head in severe unstable epilepsy
- Note: Do not use laser in patients with severe EMF sensitivity.

Eye Protection / Safety Goggles should be worn for all Class 3B and Class 4 lasers.

- Goggles MUST be worn by the patient.
- Goggles are recommended for the operator as well.
- Goggles are essential for Class 4 lasers – both patient and doctor.
- Goggles should be disinfected between each patient.

Lower power Class 2M lasers (such as visible red-light lasers with a low power divergent beam) do not require goggles for the patient or doctor.

CHAPTER 11

PBMT / LLLT versus Laser Acupuncture

These are generally best thought of as two different therapeutic approaches, with significantly different parameters.

However, there is a degree of overlap between these two therapies. They could be viewed as opposite ends of a continuum of light therapy.

It is important to appreciate the differences between these two approaches.

Laser Acupuncture

Laser acupuncture is applied specifically to acupuncture points.

These are points on the body with increased responsiveness to stimulation, and with various specific effects both locally and distally.

It works via direct neural effects locally, segmentally, distally, and systemically, and involves many of the same neurological pathways as needle acupuncture.

Laser acupuncture also has effects via Gate Control and Segmental mechanisms but does not have a DNIC effect (Diffuse Noxious Inhibitory Control) - unlike needle acupuncture which can induce DNIC.

DNIC refers to the phenomenon where "pain inhibits pain" – pain in one body site inhibits pain in another part of the body.

This is the process where neurons in the spinal cord (WDR – Wide Dynamic Range neurons) which are responsive to stimulation from one part of the body, may be inhibited by noxious stimuli (such as heat, strong pressure, or electric stimulation) applied to another remote location in the body. This inhibition originates in the brain and affects both WDR and nociceptive neurons in the dorsal horn of the spinal cord.

For laser acupuncture, very low energy doses are typically used - in the order of 0.01 – 0.5 Joule per point. Low power lasers are used - typically 1-60 mW.

The Arndt-Schulz Law is utilised. This says:

- Low doses of an intervention STIMULATE the organism
- Medium doses cause a PLATEAU EFFECT
- High doses INHIBIT the organism
- Very high doses can KILL

Laser acupuncture uses acupuncture pathways and the specific properties of acupuncture points.

It involves superficial stimulation of tissues, has an on/off "all or nothing" effect, and requires precise point location.

Laser Therapy / PBMT / LLLT

- Low Level Laser Therapy (LLLT / PBMT) treats anatomical areas of the body.

- LLLT relies on local anti-inflammatory and analgesic effects directly on body tissues.
- It relies on direct stimulation of the target tissues. Hence higher laser doses are used in the order of 1 – 10 Joules per point, with higher power lasers eg. 100mW and above
- Deeper tissues can be treated.
- The response to LLLT is dose related and requires application to correct anatomical structures.

Depth of penetration for stimulation of the acupuncture point varies between:

Superficial stimulation (laser acupuncture and Japanese acupuncture

Versus

Deeper stimulation to produce De Qi

Versus

Deep penetration into the muscle belly or teno-periosteal junction

Versus

Stimulation of the periosteum covering bone

Depending on your own model of how acupuncture works, you can aim to treat acupuncture points at any of these levels.

A-delta and C fibres have been found to send fibrils to within 5 microns of the outer surface of epidermis – this is well within the penetration depth of red-light laser (for example, the Silberbauer 1.5mW HeNe red light laser penetrates 2 – 3mm).

There are different views as to whether Infrared Laser (808nm) is needed for:

- Deep penetration into muscle

- Release of muscle spasm and myofascial trigger points

Personally, I see no need for such deep tissue penetration to get an effective acupuncture response. My aim is to treat the acupoint with ***superficial stimulation***.

However, some acupuncturists do believe that this deep tissue penetration is essential.

Empirically I have got as good results with the Silberbauer 1.5mW HeNe Laser as anyone else has achieved with any other type of acupuncture – be it superficial or deep needling, or high power 808nm Infrared Laser.

Newer red-light diode lasers (eg. Silberbauer 8mW CL Minilase) are more compact and durable, but treatment results are no better in my experience than the original Silberbauer 1.5mW HeNe laser.

I am very happy with my low power red light laser. These days this is the Silberbauer 8mW Minilase. When treating strong responders and hyper-reactors (the bulk of my practice), I add a power-reducing tip to the laser to cut the power output to 4mW, delivering 0.06 Joules to the acupuncture point at the standard treatment time of 15 seconds.

CHAPTER 12

A Personal Approach To Acupuncture

A Whole Person Perspective

As a Western medical doctor, I have also had extensive training in counselling as well as psychotherapy.

In addition, I have had many years of experience with meditation, yoga, qigong, and with a range of natural therapies. And of course, acupuncture.

I bring all this into my wholistic understanding of the human being.

It is now time to dig deeper.

So, I offer my thoughts on understanding the human being and the journey of life.

Here is a diagram to consider:

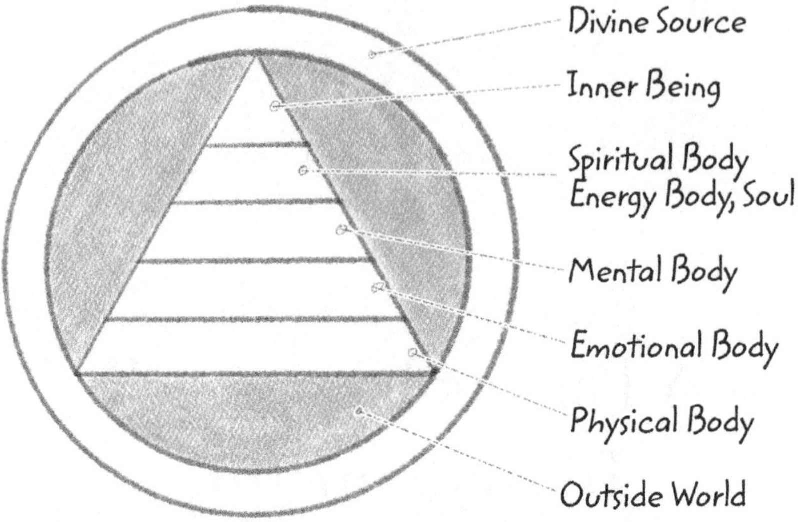

The Complete Human Being

You could see the human being as a Two-Dimensional triangle within a circle.

The triangle represents what we would normally identify as "within ourselves".

This triangle with its various divisions would therefore include the physical body, all personality aspects, and the subtle energetic and spiritual levels of ourselves.

The inner circle around the triangle represents that part of "the outside world" which in fact is ours – our own personal bit of the outer world which is a unique universe in itself, and which mirrors that which is within us.

This would include the physical and social environments, the world of nature, and the concept of Mother Nature herself.

The larger circle beyond this would represent The Divine Source that is present everywhere (in whatever way we may understand this), within which all life and creation takes place.

Alternatively, this idea can be visualised as a Three-Dimensional pyramid within a sphere.

The pyramid represents the crystalline structure of our makeup and is a shape which resonates with and amplifies life energy.

The sphere represents the totality and oneness of our world.

The Complete Human Being

There are various aspects which make up our Complete Self, including:

The Physical and Natural Environment

This includes the world of nature around us, and which can be potently nourishing and healing for us. Remember the old saying "Nature is the greatest healer."

It also includes the physical world we live in – which is often in a home and city surrounded by all sorts of pollution, stress, and busy-ness.

Traditional cultures often place great emphasis on the importance of creating and maintaining a healthy natural environment around you, in order to promote health and happiness.

The Family Environment

This is the world of our family life – our birth family, the family we may marry into, and also the family we create with a spouse and children.

It is our blood family, the ties of blood, and our inheritance.

It also includes what we inherit from our families and culture/ race – both genetic inheritance, and also family and cultural generational learning.

The Social and Cultural Environment

This is the broader society we fit into - workmates, friends, hobbies, clubs, social groups, our specific cultural and racial connections.

The Physical Body

This is the body we are most familiar with, and which is most focused on in treatment therapies – both medical and alternative/ complementary.

The physical body is certainly the earthly foundation for the whole being, and so it is always worth paying attention to getting it into good order early on in the treating and healing process. Be mindful that the goal here is about restoring good function. It is usually not necessary to aim for physical perfection – in fact such a pursuit can cause many problems, and shift the focus away from the core levels of the process which are the inner aspects of the human being.

The Emotions

This is the world of our feelings and emotional states.

It is strongly connected with our subconscious processes, and can potently control our experience of daily life.

It can create problems if we go to extremes with our emotional life – either trying to suppress our emotions, or indulging them and letting them run our lives.

The answer lies much more in finding balance and a calm centre amidst all the emotional turmoil. It is like trying to ride a wild bucking horse, and ultimately learning to guide it.

Psychological therapies, counselling, meditation, hypnotherapy, acupuncture, body therapies, yoga, various natural therapies, and healing are useful tools at this level.

The Mind

This is the world of the intellect – the rational thinking mind. Such things as logic, calculation, analysis and synthesis, concentration, and memory.

The same sorts of tools as those for the emotions are often useful here.

In addition, an emphasis on cognitive strategies, affirmations, and the physical therapies of yoga, tai chi and qigong can be particularly helpful.

The Spiritual Level

This is commonly looked at as the inner level of the person.

It used to be strictly the province of the church, but these days it is open to us all.

It is the place of the big life issues such as: Who am I? Is there a God? Is there life after death? Is there a soul? What is the point of my life? Where have I come from, and where am I going?

It is also about the search for fulfillment and meaning, connectedness and love.

It also relates to the unseen subtle levels of ourselves – our energy body or bodies, the astral body, and the soul or spirit, in whatever way these are understood by the individual. This is the realm where spiritual healing and spiritual counselling can have a potent benefit.

The Personality Self

This is the combination of bodies which together make up what we call "myself".

It is really the combination of the physical, emotional, and mental bodies, along with some aspects of the spiritual body. These add together to produce the "incarnational vehicle", the suit we wear for this lifetime on Earth. As part of this personality self, the ego or "little self" appears – the "me" of daily life experience.

Inner Being

Beyond all the other bodies, there is a place within each of us of pure consciousness, of pure awareness, the space of knowing. It is the true core of ourselves, the divine aspect of each of us. It is the space where we say "I am" from. This is the True Self.

It is the fragment of The Divine within each of us, like a precious gem waiting to be found and to be brought into the light of day to be polished and cherished.

Connecting with this Inner Consciousness is crucial. This level can override all others and important shifts at this level can result in seemingly miraculous healings, such as spontaneous remission of illness, even of such things as cancer. Allowing of course that such a healing is in accordance with the person's unique life journey and inner purpose.

In fact, you could say that the process of life is all about developing the connection with Inner Being and living it each day. This is what the ancient practice of Yoga was all about – union with The Divine, and so transcending our experience of daily life.

Healing Versus Cure/Palliation

The medical paradigm looks at defeat of disease as the goal – it is a battle between the doctor and the illness for the health and indeed life of the patient. If victory cannot be achieved, then reduction in symptoms may be acknowledged as an acceptable although second-rate alternative. It is about cure or palliation, success or failure.

This approach tends to neglect the **human being**. Too often there is a forgetting of the humanity of both the patient and the doctor in terms of ***people*** actually leading their unique lives, and having personal experiences all day, every day.

Therefore, another approach is to look at the process of therapeutic intervention, and indeed the whole of one's life, as a journey towards wholeness. This is about living as a more complete and integrated human being – in whatever way the individual person defines this. The focus becomes more about the movement toward meaning, peace and fulfilment in life. In other words, we are talking about Healing.

Wholistic Healing

For true health and for any form of therapy or healing to be truly effective, we have to pay attention to each and every aspect of the Human Being.

We need to correct any areas where there is weakness or disturbance, while we also draw on the strengths and resources held in healthy well-functioning levels of the Human Being.

And of course, we must pay careful attention to the synthesis of all these details into the totality of the wonderful unique individual Human Being.

The fundamental aim is to assist the person to fulfil their potential, to live as a conscious integrated being, and to follow their true purpose as it arises for them.

Along the way all life experiences become grist for the mill of evolving as a complete person. There are never mistakes – only experiences which enrich one's wisdom. We learn and grow through both success and failure, and through pain and suffering, as well as through love and joy.

This is true whole person healing.

CHAPTER 13

Working With Qi, Energy and Light

A Wholistic View Of Acupuncture

In the last 100 years there have been some important Western practitioners who have contributed to expanding our understanding of acupuncture as a wholistic paradigm for treating the whole person, through a synthesis of physical treatment (stimulating acupuncture points), light therapy, and working with vital energy / Qi.

These people include, but are certainly not limited to:

George Soulie de Morant

The father of acupuncture in Europe.

French ambassador to China 1900 to 1917. He saw the impressive therapeutic effects of acupuncture firsthand and studied with various masters of the art, becoming highly proficient in Chinese medicine. On his return to France, he actively promoted and taught acupuncture for many years. At first he met strong resistance, but over time a major school of acupuncture developed from his work in France, which continues to this day. This French school has strongly influenced the development of acupuncture throughout Europe.

Soulie de Morant published his magnum opus "L'Acupuncture Chinoise" (Chinese Acupuncture) in 1955 and died shortly thereafter.

He was without doubt the founder of acupuncture in Europe, a tradition with many differences to that seen in the Anglo-Saxon world.

Dr. Felix Mann

Medical Acupuncturist in London, England.

Founder of the Medical Acupuncture Society in 1959 and First President of the British Medical Acupuncture Society in 1980.

Dr. Mann was the pioneer of acupuncture in the Anglo-Saxon world.

He studied traditional acupuncture with Dr. Anton Strobl in Munich, Prof. Johannes Bischko in Vienna, Dr. Van Nha in Montpellier, and with a number of Chinese doctors in Peking, Nanking and Shanghai.

He was the first Western physician to translate a number of the ancient Chinese acupuncture texts into English and published various books on this subject from 1963 onwards.

Dr. Mann was a great observer of what worked for his patients in London and thought deeply about acupuncture.

Over time he developed a new form of Western acupuncture which he described beautifully in his last book "Reinventing Acupuncture – A New Concept of Ancient Medicine". This book has become something of a bible for me and is essential reading.

Since then, a whole school of Western scientific medical acupuncture has developed from the work of Dr. Mann.

Needless to say, the work of Dr. Mann has influenced me greatly.

Dr. Ian Schneideman

Medical Acupuncturist on the Sunshine Coast, Australia.

He was an inspired pioneer in the synthesis of Western medicine, holistic thinking, and medical acupuncture.

His book "Medical Acupuncture – Acupuncture and the Inner Healer" is a masterpiece and must-read for all aspiring medical acupuncturists. Every page breathes wisdom and understanding.

Dr. Leon Hammer

Psychiatrist and Medical Acupuncturist in Florida, USA.

Dr. Hammer studied Traditional Chinese Medicine in the early 1970's and after that practised as both a psychiatrist and acupuncturist until 1990, when he devoted himself to teaching acupuncture.

His book "Dragon Rises, Red Bird Flies: Psychology and Chinese Medicine" is a masterful synthesis of psychoanalysis with the concepts of Traditional Chinese Medicine in the understanding of people and how to help them.

Dr. Dominik Irnich

Medical Acupuncturist in Germany and head of the Munich Pain Clinic.

Dr. Irnich and his team have developed a comprehensive understanding of the human experience of chronic pain and have created a whole-person model for dealing with it. They have also carried out extensive research in the area of chronic pain. This work continues.

Dr. Irnich has edited an excellent book "Myofascial Trigger Points – Comprehensive diagnosis and treatment".

Dr. Richard Gerber

Medical specialist in internal medicine, working in Michigan, USA.

He has also trained in a range of alternative, traditional and metaphysical healing systems.

Dr. Gerber has authored a pioneering book "Vibrational Medicine" on the integration of various traditional healing systems, including acupuncture, with conventional Western medicine.

He utilises the results of scientific research where possible.

Dr. Ewald Einoder

Psychiatrist and Medical Acupuncturist in Melbourne, Australia.

Dr. Einoder sees that acupuncture is one of the few therapies which "bridge the realms". It connects the visible and the invisible, the material world with the spiritual/energetic/subtle realms.

Ewald has a great understanding of the human condition and of the many ways in which acupuncture can help.

He points out that acupuncture works NOT primarily via physical effects within the cell.

Rather it works on the energy field surrounding the cell – it effects the context within which the cell functions.

This has been found by scientists from Albert Einstein ("the sole governing principle of the particle is the field it exists within"), through to Bruce Lipton ("the sole governing force of the cell is its environment - both physical and energetic)".

Ewald is keen on the quote from Prof. Dr. Anton Jayasuriya "the person behind the needle is more important than the needle itself".

A great way to emphasize the important contribution of the consciousness and skill of the acupuncturist.

CHAPTER 14

My Approach To Acupuncture

I look at the person before me from a Whole Person Perspective and aim to find out why they are seeing me.

What is their expectation of the interaction and specifically of the treatment with me.

And can I potentially fulfil their wish.

If not, it is usually best to refer them to another practitioner more suited to help this person.

I aim to be really clear with the person about what it is reasonable to expect from our treatment program.

I take a thorough history from the person both from the Western medical and TCM acupuncture points of view. This includes information about lifestyle, diet, family, and environmental aspects. This is basically a thorough psycho-social history.

Information about past medical history and family medical history is important to look for possible patterns of illness that may be relevant.

Fundamentally, I want to find out about them as a person – "what makes them tick".

If we do agree to proceed, I always take the person through an Informed Consent process about laser acupuncture.

So, as you could imagine this all takes time. Hence a 1-hour first consultation is not unusual.

Through the interaction I aim to get a sense of who this person really is, what are their strengths that we might call on, and what are gaps or areas of deficiency we might need to attend to.

And through it all, it is most important to keep in mind what the person actually wants my help with. What is the person asking for?

Refer to the chapter "A Personal Approach To Acupuncture - A Whole Person Perspective".

Key Principles I Like To Work From

Everything has a place.

There is a place for everything – both in terms of treatment for a patient, and also in terms of life generally. Whether it be a specific dietary approach, learning to meditate, taking up Yoga, beginning a new relationship, a new job, or having a MacDonald's burger. Whatever.

It's about knowing the right thing to use, at the right time, in the right way.

Always be a Doctor, *first.*

The whole point about medical acupuncture is that it is based on Western medicine, and on the fact that you are a well-qualified experienced medical doctor. You need to know your anatomy properly and to have good procedural skills, as well as being able to consider differential diagnoses and not miss that leaking aneurysm, and to avoid possible complications such as pneumothorax from an inappropriately inserted acupuncture needle.

In acupuncture, you can never do too little.

One point only is always worth a try, especially if the patient is:

- Deeply exhausted
- Neuro-sensitised

Find the patient's "Window Of Responsiveness".

- Each person has a certain window within which they will get a positive response to an intervention from any modality.
- It is important to define the Window Of Responsiveness for each patient, at least in broad terms.
- Aim to find who needs an "atom bomb" approach versus who benefits from the "merest breath of air".
- For example, "atom bomb" approaches can include:
- Chemotherapy
- Intensive treatment with steroids or other immune suppressive medications
- Surgery
- Intensive Chinese herbal therapies

Contrast this with some examples of "merest breath of air" approaches:

- Time in Nature
- Meditation
- Subtle vibrational therapies such as flower essences, homoeopathy, and crystals

Acupuncture can cover the range from heavy-duty therapies to very subtle interventions.

Once you have a sense of the patient's "Window Of Responsiveness" then tailor your treatment to fit within this window, to get maximum benefit with minimum adverse effects.

If you over-shoot the patient's window, there is a likelihood of overloading and traumatising the patient's system and causing it to lock down. This results in an aggravation of the patient's problem, agitation, or worst of all, no response (and a subsequent possible block to other treatments as well).

If you under-shoot the window, there is too little input to trigger a response for the patient's system, and nothing happens.

This principle applies to all modalities and to all treatment systems.

"If it ain't broke, don't fix it".

If there are good responses to your treatment, don't change anything. Don't fiddle with it, try to get fancy, or add extra points.

Just keep doing the same for as long as it helps well.

Trying to "finesse" the treatment by adding that extra point in the hope of getting a better response, usually just messes things up. Don't do it!

"If it isn't working, then do something different."

This does NOT mean do more of the same, such as trying more of the same points. This will usually fail and may even aggravate the situation.

Routine western medicine is too often guilty of this. For example, if a given dose of a medication is not helping much, then let's DOUBLE the dose. This sort of approach usually worsens things.

Instead try a totally different approach – such as:

- A totally different acupoint combination.
- A different acupuncture modality.

- Or a different therapy altogether.

"The art of good medicine is to do as much nothing as possible."

From the book "The House Of God" by Dr. Samuel Shem.

A minimalist treatment approach is always a good idea – the least stimulation possible, applied without hurry, even no stimulation for a decent period of time.

Allow time for the organism to relax, open up and so have a good chance to respond well to your intervention.

This also applies to all forms of treatment from all modalities and traditions.

"Primum non nocere" – firstly do no harm.

The fundamental guiding principle of medicine – but it is too often violated in practice.

Acupuncture is one of the few treatment approaches which actually respects this dictum. (Although of course even acupuncture can be misapplied and cause harm).

The Arndt-Schulz Law

This can be a powerful ally.

You could think of it as endorsing a "homoeopathic" minimalist approach.

This law was found in older medical textbooks and its relevance is again being appreciated.

In essence it says that the gentlest lowest dose treatment that produces a good effect, is the BEST treatment.

A fuller statement of the Arndt-Schultz Law is that low doses stimulate (and that increasing the stimulus produces a better therapeutic response, up to a certain point), medium doses plateau in their effect (where increased doses do not yield any better therapeutic response), and high doses inhibit response. In fact, if the dose is taken sufficiently high enough, this can even kill the cell / organism.

This dose response follows a bell-shaped curve with the right end descending below the axis.

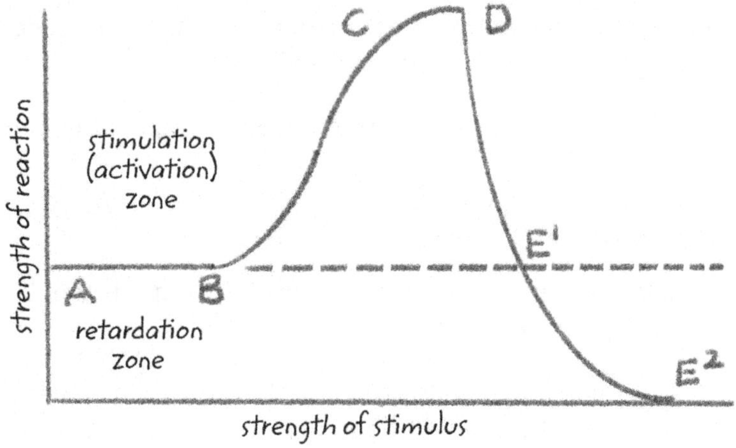

The Arndt-Schulz Law

Acupuncture tends to operate at the higher end of the "low dose phase" B-C, while Western pharmaceutical medicine and surgery tend to operate close to the plateau phase C-D, occasionally even dipping into the inhibition phase E.

This is a very important law to respect in clinical practice, whatever therapy you use.

I greatly respect and live by (as much as possible), the fundamental medical maxim of "Primum non nocere":

Firstly, do no harm.

Finally, a principle I am a great believer in:

"The art of good medicine is to do as much nothing as possible"

From "The House Of God" by Samuel Shem

Factors In Getting Good Results With Acupuncture

Good rapport between doctor and patient.

You the doctor are able to formulate a suitable acupoint prescription for the individual patient.

Review your acupoint prescription at each session based on the results of the previous treatment.

Exact palpation and stimulation of the relevant reactive acupoints.

Touch the patient gently and often (with their consent).

> This helps the patient to relax. So often the patient says "no doctor ever examined me fully like this" – this helps to inspire the patient's confidence in your work. It also allows for the recognised effect of "the doctor's healing hands" – so often described in old medical textbooks and teachings.

If you are able to, you can project Qi to the patient while touching them during the acupuncture treatment:

> This can be through specific practises from Qigong or other healing traditions, such as Reiki.
>
> It can also be done very simply by you the doctor first going into a relaxed neutral meditative state, then either blessing the patient or simply wishing them well, with no set agenda or specific outcomes in mind.

The regular practice of meditation, yoga, tai chi, or especially qigong, by you the doctor can give you a direct experience of the subtle energies the ancient acupuncture masters talked about, and it will enhance the results of your treatment for your patient. It is also good for your own general health and state of mind.

Expectations of Response to Acupuncture Treatment

In general, I suggest that you would expect to see signs of a useful response to a given point sequence within 2 – 3 treatments.

This may be specific symptom improvement, or may simply be general responses in the patient such as better vitality, improved sleep and clearer mental function.

If there is no significant improvement within 3 treatments, then you should change the acupoint combination.

In fact, with my 30+ years of experience with acupuncture, along with my training as a meditator, qigong practitioner and healer, I actually expect to see signs of improvement from each treatment. If not, I will carefully review the point combination, and probably make some changes.

Such an expectation of a positive response from each treatment really only applies for those practitioners who have become a master of their craft.

The sorts of acupoint changes may include any of:

> More points along the same lines (for example, if say Right LR3 was used initially, then try Bilateral LR3).
>
> Add a local point
>
> Add an Ear Point
>
> Try a totally new point combination – by retaking the case and re-analysing from first principles.

Acupuncture Points With Powerful Autonomic Effects

My colleague Dr. Tim Begbie rightly emphasizes the **autonomic** effects of acupuncture as being very important. There is excellent autonomic innervation of superficial blood vessels at the hands, wrists, ankles, and feet. Acupoints at these sites are easily accessible and so give good access to autonomic modulation.

These points can be very useful in various conditions with significant associated autonomic instability or dysfunction.

The autonomic nervous system is made up of the sympathetic ("fight or flight") and parasympathetic ("rest and digest" and "feed and breed") nervous systems.

The points include:

> The classic "homoeostatic points": LI4, LI11, ST36, SP6, GV20 ("meeting point of 100 points" therefore balancing), and some people would include LR3
>
> Specific autonomic points (typically at wrists and ankles where there are superficial blood vessels with associated autonomic innervation, close to the body surface): LU9, PC6, HT7, ST36, BL62, (also LI4, SP6, LR3, KI3), and the Ear Points – Shenmen, Sympathetic.
>
> There is a sequence of points with innervation from the sympathetic nervous system which emerge from the thoracic and lumbar spine from levels T1 to L3.
>
> These sympathetic points include the Huatuojiaji points and the points on the inner arm of the Bladder channel (BL11 to BL23) at these spinal levels T1-L3. These points can have a useful effect on the related spinal segment.
>
> Sympathetic tone to the head, neck and heart can be stimulated by acupuncture to the cervical sympathetic chain (arising from the upper thoracic sympathetic outflow) using points TE17, SI17, ST11. TE17 and SI17 are adjacent to the superior cervical sympathetic ganglion at the C2 spinal level. ST11 is adjacent to the inferior cervical sympathetic/

stellate ganglion at the C7 level of the neck. Great care must be used with needling these points because they are adjacent to vulnerable structures, but laser is fine.

In addition, there are parasympathetic nerves emerging in the sacrum from S2-S4 which have powerful effects on the pelvic viscera as well as on nerve and blood vessel function in the legs (hence can be used for vascular intermittent claudication and for claudication due to spinal canal stenosis).

Useful parasympathetic points include BL32 to BL34 over the sacrum.

The vagus nerve arises from parasympathetic outflow in the brainstem and has widespread effects on many organs within the chest and abdomen. In addition, cranial nerves II, VII, IX and X arise from brainstem parasympathetic outflow.

Points such GV26, TE17, GB34, ST36, SP6 and Earpoints Shenmen, Vagus, and the Zero Point, can have powerful vagal effects.

You can use any or all of the points in these sequences in an individual patient at any given time.

Graded Progression In "Tonifying Treatment"

These are points used to boost core vitality – from gentlest to strongest:

A "Tonifying Sequence" as described by Geoff Greenbaum and Anton Jayasuriya is GV14, LI4, ST36, SP6 (+/- LR3). This includes the "Three Great Points": LI4, ST36, SP6 – so called because these points are very powerful and have so many effects (have a look at their functions from both the TCM and "Western physiological" points of view).

If no benefit, add CV6 (Qihai - "The Sea Of Energy") to the above Tonifying Sequence.

If no response, next change to trying the Yuan Source Point of the key disturbed organ noted on your case analysis.

Next try the Yuan Source Point of the Kidney (KI3). This is tonifying the Essential Kidney Qi.

Next try the Back-Shu Point of Kidney (BL23) PLUS Mingmen (GV4 – "The Gate Of Life"). This is stronger tonifying of the Essential Kidney Qi.

Finally try the most potent method for tonifying the Essential Kidney Qi by treating the two endpoints of the Kidney meridian – KI27 and KI1.

And if all else fails, try Prayer. I kid you not. Miracles have on occasion occurred from such things.

General Guidelines For Laser Acupuncture versus Needle Acupuncture:

You will find me repeating these key points during the text.

So here we go.

For laser acupuncture, in general you need to use 50% more local points PLUS bilateral distal points, compared to needle acupuncture.

You must also be exact about finding the reactive acupuncture point.

However, you must of course respect the individuality of the patient and so vary this rule of thumb according to the needs and responsiveness of the individual patient - sometimes even down to just 1 point treated for 1 second in a very sensitive patient.

Principles of Treatment

Hyperacute conditions – use 1 suitable distal point on the

first day, and treat daily until settled – for example, for acute locked back use GV26. After the first day or so if the patient is responding well, you may then treat as if it is an Acute Condition (see next below).

Acute conditions – use several local + distal points, and in general treat every 2 to 3 days until settled.

With Hyper Acute and Acute Conditions, it may be worthwhile having a "booster treatment" about 1 week after the condition settles.

Chronic conditions – use distal / reflex acupoints only at first, and treat much less frequently, often every 1 to 4 weeks.

Then as treatment progresses carefully add 1 or points at a time, if relevant.

Finally, one or two local points might be used (and quite often might never be used), once the patient's central sensitisation has settled and in essence they have become a "normal responder".

Strong Responders and Hyper-Reactors

Some patients (perhaps 1 in 5) are far more responsive to treatment inputs than the average patient. These Strong Responder patients constitutionally have a magnified and healthy response to acupuncture. Hence treat them very gently – often just 1 or 2 well-chosen points with minimal or no stimulation. Also treat them much less frequently (perhaps once every 2 – 4 weeks initially to allow time for their treatment response to fully unfold before treating them again). The old maxim applies very well here – "a little bit goes a long way".

This concept is based on the pioneering work of Dr. Felix Mann – see "Strong Responders" in the section about Dr. Felix Mann.

In some ways the sensitivity of Strong Responders may seem similar to "centrally sensitised" patients, but without all the aggravations and poor treatment response often seen in these sensitised patients.

In fact, these "Hyper-Reactor" sensitised patients are very unhealthy and have come to this state through a long history of adverse life events, sicknesses and problems leading to a very depleted state. Often, they have a significant Kidney Qi deficiency, or at least a severely aggravated Liver or Spleen syndrome. These are often the patients who present with a difficult-to-treat chronic pain syndrome such as pain amplification syndrome, fibromyalgia, or RSD.

See the section about treatment of patients with CFS / Fibromyalgia.

These Hyper-Reactor patients are often the ones where it can be said of them "easy to aggravate, but hard to help".

Neuro-Sensitisation

This is a phenomenon which can occur in some pain situations.

In essence the painful area becomes overly sensitive to stimuli so that normal touch or minimally painful stimuli are felt as significantly painful.

This process is neurologically mediated due to specific nociceptive (pain) nerve fibres becoming overly sensitive to inputs. There are various mechanisms for this to occur.

Peripheral Sensitisation is where nerves in the area of the pain become over-sensitive due to local release of inflammatory mediators.

Central Sensitisation is the process where this increased sensitivity is due to changes centrally in the brain and spinal cord in the nociceptive pain pathways. The original pain-inducing trauma has ceased, but the pain experience continues due to these central changes. These central neurological changes are referred to as "neuro-plasticity".

Hyperalgesia is the phenomenon where painful stimuli are felt at much greater intensities of pain.

Allodynia is the phenomenon where even minimal non-painful stimuli produce significant pain.

Central Sensitisation often causes the area of pain to greatly expand in size, sensitivity, intensity, and chronicity.

Central Sensitisation is much trickier to treat, whether by conventional medicine or by acupuncture, although acupuncture often has an important role to play in managing a person in this situation.

Neuro-Sensitisation is well discussed in the books:

> "Pain – The person, the science, the clinical interface" edited by Patricia Armati and Roberta Chow. IP Communications. Melbourne. 2015
>
> "An Introduction To Western Medical Acupuncture" edited by Adrian White, Mike Cummings and Jacqueline Filshie. 2nd Edition. Churchill Livingstone Elsevier. 2018
>
> "Medical Acupuncture – A Western Scientific Approach" edited by Jacqueline Filshie, Adrian White and Mike Cummings. 2nd Edition. Elsevier. 2016

Fast Reactors, Slow Reactors, and Average Responders

These terms are pretty much self-explanatory.

A Fast Reactor

Is someone who gets virtually immediate and dramatic responses to acupuncture treatment. These patients are usually very gratifying to treat, but beware of doing too much and over-stimulating them. This group overlaps significantly with Strong Responders.

A Slow Reactor

Is a person where everything happens very slowly. It can take a number of treatments to see any real changes, many points may need to be used (relative to an Average or Strong Responder), and improvement often occurs in small increments over time.

Average Responders

Obviously are somewhere in the middle between these two extremes, and they make up the bulk of the population.

The Acupuncture Non-Responder

It is true to say that a few people do not respond to acupuncture treatment.

There is always the fundamental principle that the doctor must be competent at their chosen modality of acupuncture. If acupuncture is not applied competently then do not expect decent treatment results – instead the doctor should go back to school and improve their acupuncture techniques.

Another fundamental principle or sine qua non, is that the doctor has established suitable rapport with the patient, and a therapeutic relationship has been developed. I cannot over-emphasize the importance of this. It comes from the doctor having suitable counselling skills (be it from training or just natural aptitude), and an overall empathy with the patient. It is actually fundamental to all healing, and it is rare for benefit to occur for the patient without basic rapport and trust between doctor and patient.

Sometimes this lack of acupuncture response is related to some active underlying pathology (physical, emotional, or psycho-social) which is not being addressed. Once this problem is uncovered and then attended to, the patient will usually then begin to respond to treatment.

On occasion the problem is the chosen acupuncture treatment modality itself – there are a few people who do better (or will only respond to) one particular modality, be it needles (as a refinement superficial versus deep needling), red light laser, or infra-red laser. But in my experience, this is only rarely the issue.

I would say that usually the issue is choosing a suitable point combination, and having the flexibility to revise the treatment plan and change the points should there be inadequate response in the expected timeframe. The chosen point prescription on occasion may need to be reviewed or changed at every individual treatment.

Having said all this there are indeed a few people who truly are acupuncture non-responders – in my estimation, no more than 10% of the population, probably much less.

There are various theories as to the reason for this Non-Responder Status – proposals include genetic predisposition, dysfunction of the autonomic nervous system, imbalanced dopamine levels in the CNS, or chronically low serotonin levels in the brain. Any of these options may apply on occasion.

However, I have observed that there are some psychological factors that typically apply in these Non-Responders:

A very rigid state of mind, that admits no possibility of actual change

Chronic levels of tension, both mentally and physically – this equates to a state of chronic hyper-arousal

A generally pessimistic / depressive attitude to life, often coupled with a desperate search for "the cure", and a clinging on to the doctor as their last hope in life.

This sort of patient is often "overly intellectual" and prizes their rational thinking brain above all else. To my way of thinking, these people are often "stuck in their heads and have closed their hearts".

In my view nothing can be done for these patients – unless in their own time they come to a psychological space where they are truly available to change and to embrace the flow of Life.

And I would say this typically only occurs once the person has had some sort of spiritual experience which opens them to the possibility of something greater and wiser than themselves – some would call this "finding God".

In this regard the 12 Step Program of Alcoholics Anonymous has something to offer.

It could be said that these psychologically rigid Non-Responders are addicted to their pain and suffering, and the only way through this is total surrender to something greater than themselves.

Differences between Illness Patterns and Acupuncture Response based on Genetics

My impression is that the different racial groups have significant differences in the patterns of illness they present with, and the different styles and point combinations they typically respond to.

I think genetics may be important in these differing patterns.

Caucasians

The so-called "white races" such as Anglo-Saxons and Celts, Scandinavians, and Germanic races.

These groups tend to follow the patterns observed by Dr. Felix Mann and recorded in his book "Reinventing Acupuncture".

There is a preponderance of Liver disorders in these people, but there may also be Spleen/Stomach, Kidney or Lung disturbances on occasion.

These groups give rise to the observation of the significant incidence of Strong Responders and Hyper-Reactors.

A number of these people are unusually and highly responsive to acupuncture treatment, and so a little bit goes a long way. Strong Responders.

In addition, some of these people are highly depleted and so have low vitality with a "low Qi state". Life has been rough with them. These are the Hyper-Reactors who aggravate easily but are hard to help. People with all sorts of chronic degenerative or auto-immune conditions – MS, CFS, Fibromyalgia, SLE, multi-system disease, etc.

LR3 is a keystone of treatment for many of these people.

You may also need to deal with Spleen, Kidney or Lung issues.

And of course, Stress!

Hence points such as LR3, LR8, SP6, KI3, GV15, GV20, HT7, and PC6 are commonly used. And start treatment very gently with only 1 or 2 distal points – no local points at first, except for acute localised illness/trauma.

It may well be that we are seeing here the effects of Western "civilised living". Too much pollution, living out of balance with nature, poor diet, medication overuse, drug abuse, and stress from all sorts of angles. Really messes up the human being. And epigenetics suggests these disorders can be inherited – as we often do see in practice.

Mediterranean races

This includes people from Italy, Greece, Spain and France.

The typical patterns of illness are very similar to those of Caucasians – except perhaps Liverish diseases are even more predominant.

Treat as for Caucasians. Remember the value of LR3 +/- LR8.

Chinese origin

People with a Chinese genetic background seem to commonly present with Stomach / Spleen disorders. They typically respond well to the classic TCM approach developed over an extended period of time in China. No surprise of course.

Usual treatment would involve lots of local points, possibly with the addition of a few distal points. Many needles used. Fine if there is pain or even bleeding from needling.

The impression is to use robust acupuncture treatment for robust constitutions. This seems to be at the opposite end of the spectrum to many Caucasian and Mediterranean people.

Indian subcontinent

This includes people from Pakistan, Bangladesh, Sri Lanka and of course India itself. It also includes Indians who migrated to other countries, whether it be that they currently migrated or it was their ancestors who left the homeland.

These people are also very prone to Liverish diseases, but as Prof. Anton Jayasuriya pointed out, care must be taken with direct treatment of the Liver. Anton generally avoided use of LR3 as he felt it was too strong – there was a significant risk of people aggravating, or dropping their blood pressure and fainting.

Hence LR8 (the HeSea point) is often a better option for these people. Treat them very gently at first, maybe even totally avoid Liver points initially.

Middle Eastern

I have had much less experience with people from this region, but my tentative impression is that they are a combination of Indian and Chinese patterns in their response to acupuncture, tending more towards the Chinese patterns the closer their genetic origins are to China.

You could say they seem to have a combination of Liver and Spleen/Stomach disorders.

Africans

I have had little experience treating people from Africa, and so can make few comments. I just treat any such people from first principles and in my usual way, proceed very gently with treatment.

I would point out that those Africans whose ancestors originally came from Europe do of course share the same illness and acupuncture response patterns as their European forebears.

All of this needs to be properly researched.

Perhaps this is something you may wish to take up and research more fully.

For patients with CFS or Fibromyalgia

My experience is that:

> These patients easily aggravate or are "overloaded" by treatments, including acupuncture.
>
> You must find the patient's "**Individual Window Of Responsiveness**" in terms of both suitable modality and intensity of treatment.
>
> If the patient is treated too "heavily" then their system cannot integrate the input and instead goes into "shock" with either a treatment aggravation (which may be severe, extended and disabling) or there is no response or at all (and this may compromise further treatments).
>
> ***The key is to use a minimum number of points applied very gently.***
>
> That way there is a real chance of useful improvement

occurring gradually over time.

In general, do not focus on individual symptoms initially, instead try to treat whatever is the **fundamental disturbance** in the patient.

Perhaps this may be Stress / Emotional Disturbance, or Immune Deficiency, or a key disordered organ / meridian – often this will be "Kidney Deficiency".

An overall approach for treating patients with very depleted vitality, chronic fatigue, CFS or fibromyalgia:

Work gently on slowly rebuilding their Qi (lifeforce) before giving specific attention to individual problems and symptoms.

For example, you could treat one key point every 3 to 4 weeks – such as GV20 or KI3 (Yuan Source point for the Kidney – to boost Kidney Qi). Perhaps even both points together in due course.

Once there is a decent improvement in vitality and sleep, then you can slowly add a few additional points to tackle any specific residual problems, such as pain in discrete areas.

Therefore, typically begin treatment with 1 or 2 points chosen from:

An Ear Point for the key process

A simple emotionally balancing / tranquillising point – such as GV15 or GV20 alone

A point used very gently for the disturbed organ – beware this may cause an aggravation, so use very cautiously, or perhaps not at the first treatment if unsure just how sensitive the patient is. Typically, this will be a Yuan Source Point or HeSea Point - such as KI3 (or KI10), or LR3 (or LR10), or SP6.

CHAPTER 15

Treatment Of Specific Chronic Complex Conditions

Chronic Fatigue Syndrome (CFS)

Definition of CFS

CFS is defined as ongoing fatigue for greater than 6 months in association with some or all of:

- Sleep disturbance
- Daytime drowsiness
- Muscle and joint pains
- Headaches
- Recurring fevers
- Swollen lymph nodes
- Abdominal disturbance (constipation, diarrhoea, bloating, flatulence)
- Emotional disturbance (anxiety, depression)
- Cognitive disturbance (confusion, poor memory, difficulty

with word finding, poor concentration)

Basic causes of CFS

Stress and distress

Sleep deprivation

Dysfunctional coping mechanisms (pain avoidance) leading to perpetuation of distress, including:

- Workaholic – Busyness
- Addictions – Food, cigarettes, drugs, sport
- Depression

Triggers of CFS

Acute stress – physical, emotional, mental

Acute infection

Post - infection syndrome (viral, bacterial, fungal)

Chronic infection (such as Mycoplasma, Lyme Disease)

Candidiasis

Chemical / Drug toxicity

Heavy Metal toxicity

Food and chemical sensitivities

Adrenal Exhaustion from long-term stress

Nutritional deficiencies

Management of CFS

Rest

Restoration of good sleep

Graduated exercise. This must be done in a fluid way responsive to the individual patient's needs of the time.

Relaxation therapy

Counselling – identify and correct dysfunctional patterns and their underlying causes

Simplify one's life and attend to core needs

Qigong

Nutritional support

Herbal / homoeopathic support

Chelation for Heavy Metal Toxicity

Anti-fungal / anti-microbial therapy

Acupuncture

Acupuncture for CFS

Clinical Syndromes

Liver Excess:

Depression / irritability

Muscle pains and headaches

Allergies

Food / chemical sensitivities

Chemical / drug toxicity

Heavy metal toxicity

Chronic infections and post-infection syndrome

Spleen Deficiency:

Obsessive thinking – chronically worrying about their health

Patient is overall "Very Heavy" – physically, mentally, emotionally

Candidiasis

Gastro-Intestinal disturbance - bloating, chronic diarrhoea or constipation, leaky gut syndrome

Menstrual disturbances

Kidney Qi Deficiency:

Chronic anxiety

"Weak and wobbly"

Pains everywhere

Neurasthenia

Adrenal exhaustion

Congenital Kidney Qi deficiency from intra-uterine problems or major childhood diseases

Practical tips in treatment for CFS

Acupuncture response requires energy in the system to work with.

Therefore, if the patient is totally depleted:

> **First** instill some energy with restoration of good sleep, Qigong, herbs, homoeopathy, or Intravenous Vitamin C
>
> **Then** use acupuncture to rebalance the person

A strong responder will **always** get some benefit from acupuncture

So always let a good responder have a trial of acupuncture

It is also worth trying a few gentle treatments if the patient's responsiveness profile is unknown

Patients with CFS are often Strong Responders

Therefore, begin with only 1 or 2 points, and use minimal stimulation

Treat infrequently (for example every 2 - 4 weeks)

Less is always better (especially if treatment is difficult)

Beware the Hyper-reactor (very difficult to treat successfully)

Hyper - Reactors

These patients have a very difficult combination of over-responsiveness to treatment with markedly depleted Kidney Qi

Treat very gently (for example treat 1 point for a few seconds only and treat very occasionally - every 3 to 6 weeks)

Focus on boosting Kidney Qi first, or on one sedative/balancing point (for example GV20 only)

Point combinations – Often used for CFS

These are all potential points but only a few would be selected depending on patient factors:

GV20

GV15

Tranquilising Sequence - GV15 + LI4 + PC6 + H7 +/- HT3

LR3

SP6

KI3

CV6 + SP6 + LR3

For Gastro-Intestinal disturbance - CV12, CV6, ST36, ST25, BL25

ST40 can be useful for catarrh and mucus over-production (excess phlegm)

For chronic allergies, choose from LR3, SP6, SP10, LI11, GV14 Ear - allergy point

For generalised widespread musculo-skeletal pain try the combination of GV14 +TE5 + GB34

For extreme fatigue try:

KI3

KI3 + LR3

KI3 + KI5 + KI7

GV4 + BL20 + BL23

PC6 + TE5 (open the Inner Gate and Outer Gate to allow harmonization of Qi flow between deep and superficial levels)

KI27

Ear points can include any or all of:

Shenmen

Liver

Spleen

Kidney

Allergy

Zang-Fu (aspirin point on Darwin's tubercle)

Chronic Musculo-Skeletal Pain and Fibromyalgia

Acute Musculo-Skeletal Pain typically commences with acute tissue trauma.

A localized classic physiological healing response takes place – inflammation leads to granulation tissue leads to resolution.

The process is self-limiting – it leads to either:

- Resolution / healing (with or without residual scarring)
- Death

However, in some situations the problem may persist and lead to ***Chronic*** Musculo-Skeletal Pain.

There are 5 types of Chronic Musculo-Skeletal Pain:

Local Ongoing Physical Pathology

There is an ongoing tissue irritant causing ongoing inflammation and pain.

Important to check for ongoing causes of pathology – such as cancer, rheumatoid arthritis

Local Reflex Muscle Spasm

No objective signs of pathology or inflammation.

The original trauma has now healed – but has led to local chronic muscle spasm. This is due to the original traumatic pain setting off ongoing activation of Lower Motor Neurons in the local area (ongoing local spinal segmental activation of the Dorsal Motor Neurons) combined with CNS activation

Treatment – Usually responds quickly and well to acupuncture focusing on treating pain with local points.

Fibromyalgia

The original trauma has now healed – but has led to:

Central Nervous System (CNS) sensitization with whole-body pain amplification syndrome

Whole person response to pain

Sensitivity of soft tissues throughout the body

Often there is associated fatigue, insomnia, mood changes (typically depression), and cognitive changes such as poor concentration

In essence, we see a local injury which leads to a neuro-sensitisation process. As a result, the traumatised area becomes swollen and tender (greater than and out of proportion to the injury). The swelling is due to axon leakage in the area of pain.

Fibromyalgia may progress to **Regional Pain Syndrome.**

Aggravating Factors for development of Regional Pain Syndrome are:

Nature of the original physical trauma

Underlying psychological trauma – especially childhood abuse

Medications – Lyrica and Gabapentin

Depression

Psychological "catastrophising"

Compensation / Workcover issues

Sleep deprivation

Hormones (excess oestrogen state)

Treatment:

Responds well to minimalist acupuncture, treating a few key constitutional points. Need to treat over a long period of time

– often 2 years

Restore good sleep

Gentle graduated mobilization – at a pace which suits the individual patient

Qigong is often very helpful

Regional Pain Syndrome

Also known as CRPS – Chronic Regional Pain Syndrome.

Sympathetic nervous system changes occur.

The original trauma (now healed) is followed by reflex sympathetic changes:

Regional skin hypersensitivity

Allodynia = non-painful stimulus such as light touch provokes pain response

Hyperaesthesia = mild painful stimulus such as pressure to tendon evokes severe pain response

Excess skin sweating

Local trauma / pain leads to neuro-sensitisation of Wide Dynamic Range Neurons (WDR) in the spinal cord. As a result, these WDR neurons are turned up to maximum producing ongoing CNS activation (activation of thalamus).

In essence local pain / trauma leads to CNS Activation.

Treatment:

Responds slowly to gentle acupuncture with 1 – 2 general balancing CNS points (eg. GV20 alone).

May eventually suddenly improve.

Regional Pain Syndrome may sometimes progress to **RSD** –

Reflex Sympathetic Dystrophy.

This is a progressed version of the reflex sympathetic changes of CRPS.

Vascular and sympathetic changes now occur in the local area of pain – producing local puffiness and cold blue skin.

Atrophy of skin and subdermal tissues, and sometimes of muscle, may occur in the long term.

Very hard to treat successfully.

Sports Injury

Localised physical trauma to muscle in a well person.

This produces local inflammation in proportion to the injury.

Treatment: Responds quickly and well to acupuncture.

Specifics of Acupuncture Treatment for Fibromylagia

Look at the whole person – physical, emotional / psychological, environmental, social.

Use a multi-modality team approach.

Acupuncture (especially used gently) often has a valuable contribution.

Remember to keep your points to the minimum necessary.

As a rule of thumb at the First Treatment **avoid local points** – use 1 or 2 well-chosen distal points or ear points.

This reduces the risk of significantly aggravating Strong Responders and Hyper Reactors – a common issue in chronic pain patients.

Chronic Conditions are generally treated every 1 to 4 weeks.

You may just use a few well-chosen distal or ear points throughout the whole treatment sequence and get very good results.

Adjust the acupoints used according to the patient's response.

Usually you need to treat slowly and gently over time.

Some patients do **ultimately** need treatment of **specific local trigger points** to get a complete result.

Always consider other factors that may need treating – such as psychological factors.

If the patient gets a good response for a few days after each treatment then repeatedly relapses after a set period of time, consider hidden pathology (psychological, family / social / cultural, or physical – including occult malignancy).

Dr. Geoff Greenbaum considered that the art of acupuncture was the treatment of ***reactive points*** on the body surface, and knowing which of these reactive points to treat on a given day.

Geoff saw the prime effect of acupuncture as homoeostatic.

In a tricky patient, Geoff considered Tranquillising Points (such as any of GV15, GV20, LI4, PC6, HT7 or Ear Shenmen) were always worth a try – either combined with a few other points, or just on their own.

Needling can be superficial or deep, gentle or strong – as long as DeQi is elicited. Laser is particularly useful because it is so gentle.

Dr. Felix Mann specialised in treating the patient very gently with just 1 needle.

It is wisely said that the master acupuncturist uses 1 point only.

As noted previously, it is best to work gently on slowly rebuilding the patient's Qi (lifeforce) before giving specific attention to individual problems and symptoms.

For example, you could treat one key point every 3 to 4 weeks

– such as **GV20** or **KI3** (Yuan Source point for the Kidney – to boost Kidney Qi). Perhaps even both points together in due course.

Once there is a decent improvement in vitality and sleep, then you can slowly add a few additional points to tackle any specific residual problems, such as pain in discrete areas.

Therefore, typically begin treatment with 1 or 2 points chosen from:

An Ear Point for the key process

A simple emotionally balancing / tranquillising point – such as GV15 or GV20 alone

A point can be used very gently for the disturbed organ – beware this may cause an aggravation, so use very cautiously, or perhaps **not** at the first treatment if unsure just how sensitive the patient is.

Typically, this will be a Yuan Source Point or HeSea Point - such as KI3 (or KI10), or LR3 (or LR10), or SP6.

Rheumatoid Arthritis

This approach also applies to treatment for other auto-immune inflammatory conditions such as SLE (lupus).

In general, these patients often have a tricky combination of

Advanced Liver Syndrome

Strong Responder – or more usually Hyper-Reactor

Many of the factors and issues around treating people with CFS also apply here.

In general start treatment with 1 or 2 well-chosen distal points.

Initially avoid local points.

Can easily aggravate – so treat very gently and infrequently, until reactivity settles to more normal levels.

Typically, these people have a Liver Syndrome – so LR3 is often very useful. In fact, LR3 may be the only point used initially.

The more active the rheumatoid arthritis and the higher the inflammatory markers are, the more gently you should treat the patient – fewer points, distal points only, and treat less frequently.

As the patient's condition improves and hopefully the inflammation reduces, the more you can start to carefully treat locally with a few points.

Remember the value of ear points to treat these patients.

You might for example start treatment with just LR3 (the Yuan Source Point for the Liver)

Then over time you might add some further anti-inflammatory points, and/or ear points corresponding to the worst areas of pain.

You could also add analgesic points.

Finally, you might add a few local points, especially as the inflammation settles.

A possible treatment sequence might be:

LR3 (or the HeSea point LR8)

Then LR3 + any of GV14 / LI4 / LI11 / ST36 / SP6 **(anti-inflammatory points)**

Or LR3 + LI4 / ST44 **(analgesic points)**

Then LR3 (+/- analgesic / anti-inflammatory points) + **Ear Points**

Then LR3 (+/- analgesic / anti-inflammatory points +/- Ear Points) + **Local Points**

As with all chronic conditions, psychological aspects may be significant whether primary or secondary to the disease.

Therefore, a **relaxation sequence** (GV15, GV20, PC6, HT7, etc) is always worth a try.

Remember to go slowly and carefully with treatment, especially with the more inflamed patients.

Multiple Sclerosis

Many of the observations about treatment of Rheumatoid Arthritis also apply here.

Psychological factors, whether primary or secondary to the disease process, are often of great importance in the general management and in acupuncture treatment, for these patients.

Hence **Relaxation Points** (Tranquillising Sequence) are often of great value.

Remember these patients are often Strong Responders or Hyper-Reactors.

The **Liverish type** may have a more **active or aggressive disease** process, and often **anger** is evident in the person. Tongue and Pulse changes will often back up this Liver condition.

The **Kidney deficient type** is often more depleted from a long history with the disease, and may be something of a burnt-out end phase of MS. The disease is often much less active, but may have deep fatigue and chronic widespread symptoms of the disease process. This sort of person may well fit the "generally weak and wobbly" description of people with chronic Kidney deficiency.

Sometimes the person will initially be a Liverish type, then as the disease progresses and becomes deeply ingrained but often less active, the pattern may change to more of a Kidney type, or at least a mixed Liver/Kidney pattern.

As with the other chronic complex conditions, treatment should follow the overall approach of treat gently and slowly, initially with only a few distal / ear points.

Some relaxation points will often be useful at some point during treatment. For example, GV15, GV20.

BL62 is often useful, as the unofficial Influential Point for the Nervous System (both central and peripheral nervous system).

Tonifying the Kidneys will often be very useful especially for the burnt-out Kidney deficient type. Points such as KI3, GV4, BL23 may be very helpful to support the Kidney energy.

LR3 and/or LR8 are often of importance in the more active Liverish type.

Ultimately you may need to add a few analgesic points (LI4, ST44), one or two anti-inflammatory points, ear points, or even the odd local point for specific pains and problems.

A possible treatment sequence might be:

GV20

Then GV20 + BL62

Then LR3 or KI3 – on its own or with GV20/BL62

Then add ear points

Finally add any relevant specific / local points (sparingly)

Be mindful that if a given point combination gives helpful results, keep repeating this combination until benefit tails off.

Chronic Neurological Conditions

In these conditions we often need to use a lot of points in treatment – as opposed to treatment of MS.

Of course, you would initially start with just a few points as always. But be prepared to increase the points extensively over time, if needed.

In general response takes time and gradual improvement is often seen over many months. It is always worth trying 6 treatments or so in conditions such as Parkinson's Disease, post-CVA (stroke), post head injury, neuropathy in all its manifestations, in fact any chronic neurological condition.

You can sometimes get very gratifying responses over time, especially if you are patient and think about what you are doing at each treatment.

Depending on the condition, we may choose from:

Cerebrally active points – GV15, GV20, Yintang. In fact, any points on the head over the brain.

Scalp Acupuncture – choose specific scalp lines depending on the condition. Often, we would start with the Motor Line in conditions of weakness / paraplegia / paralysis, or with the Sensory Line in conditions primarily characterised by sensory distortion.

BL62 – as the unofficial Influential Point for the nervous system, both central and peripheral.

An Influential Point for muscles, tendons and ligaments may be useful – GB34 or LR3.

We often use points along the affected limbs – usually on the extensor Yang body surface. Groups of points such as:

LI4 / LI11 / LI15

TE5 / TE10 / TE14

GB30 / GB34 / GB40 or 41

ST36 / ST41 / ST44

Other local points can be added as indicated over time.

CHAPTER 16

Important Recent Developments In Acupuncture (post-WWII)

Acupuncture is a living and progressing art/science, and there have been a number of significant developments since 1950.

Dr. Felix Mann's periosteal points. This was originally done with very deep needling and strong manual stimulation to reactive points on the periosteum of bones in the area of pain. It has since been found that, due to the multi-level projection of nerve fibrils related to an acupuncture point, these points can be effectively stimulated with standard acupuncture methods (needling or laser) at any depth.

Tim-Mee point for tobacco smoking addiction. This point was described by American psychiatrist/acupuncturist Dr James Olms in 1981. The point is located 1 cun from LU7 on the dorsal aspect of the wrist (near TE5), and it is typically tender and swollen in a smoker.

Note – Often effective treatment for smokers is:

Tim-Mee + GV15/GV20 + "constitutional point" for the key TCM organ disturbance (eg. LR3 or SP6)

Possible addition of CV17 and Ear Shenmen / Lung for COPD

Possible addition of a more extended tranquillising sequence if stress/anxiety/depression is an issue – points such as LI4, PC6, HT7, HT3, Ear Shenmen

Treat weekly for 4 weeks then review at 1 month and 3 months

Ear Acupuncture

First developed in the 1950's in both China and independently in France by Dr. Paul Nogier. This micro-system acupuncture is based on the fact that the ear has intensive vagal innervation. The vagus nerve has a very broad distribution to many organs, and so enables a widespread range of effects from ear acupuncture. Can be done effectively with needles or laser.

More recent developments with ear acupuncture include:

The NADA protocol for drug addiction developed in 1985 by Dr Michael Smith in New York. The typical sequence is bilateral Lung, Liver, Kidney, Shenmen, Sympathetic/Autonomic.

"Battlefield acupuncture" developed by Dr Richard Niemtzow in the USA in 2001 for soldiers with acute pain and distress/trauma. The typical sequence is Cingulate Gyrus, Thalamus, Omega 2, Shenmen, Zero Point.

As an extension of "battlefield acupuncture", Dr Joseph Helms developed the Auricular Trauma Protocol (ATP) for PTSD (post-traumatic stress disorder) which has seen effective results. The sequence is Hypothalamus, Amygdala, Hippocampus, Master Cerebral, Zero Point, Shenmen. In practice you can just use several of these points with good effect. I rather like Shenmen, Zero Point, +/- Master Cerebral points for PTSD.

Scalp Acupuncture

Based on the surface projections of anatomical regions of the brain cortex. Developed in the 1970's in China. Can be performed effectively with needles or laser. Often useful for:

Head injury recovery from trauma or CVA (stroke)

Parkinson's Disease management

Sometimes used for resistant chronic pain

Often combined with "cerebrally active" acupoints such as GV14, GV15, GV20, Yintang, other tender points on the GV channel on the scalp, and BL62 (as the unofficial influential point for the central nervous system)

Autonomic Effects

The understanding of the importance of Autonomic Dysfunction in many conditions, and that well-applied acupuncture can have powerful therapeutic autonomic effects.

Fascia

The recent understanding of the importance of Fascia and Fascial Planes in the function of the human body, and that acupuncture may, in part, work via fascial effects. The fascia has specific planes of connection (some of which mirror certain acupuncture meridians), and it carries an electrical charge – this may be relevant to transmission of impulses along meridians in response to specific stimulation of certain acupuncture points.

Acupuncture continues to evolve. It is certainly not a fixed and ossified method, as ancient texts or TCM may sometimes imply.

CHAPTER 17

Aspects of TCM in my practice

Understanding the Essence of the TCM Organs

I find it useful to understand the fundamental principles on which each TCM Organ functions.

Solid Yin organs house and store the deep energy of the element.

Hollow Yang organs transport the energy of the element.

I see the essence of each Element as:

> **WOOD** (Liver / Gallbladder) = WILL (especially WILL In Action)
>
> **FIRE** (Heart / Small Intestine, Pericardium / Triple Energiser)
>
> > **Fire of life.** = Creative inspiration. Consciousness.
> >
> > **Heart** = Core emotions, the seat of the Soul

Pericardium = Membrane covering of the heart = protection of one's deep innermost feelings

Triple Energiser = The three body cavities (thorax, abdomen, pelvis) = the principle of Homoeostasis

EARTH (Spleen / Stomach) = NOURISHMENT (mothering, digestion physically and mentally, hormonal system, gastro-intestinal tract)

METAL (Lung / Large Intestine) = RELEASE, DETACHMENT & RENEWAL. Letting go of attachments, and finding oneself.

WATER (Kidney / Bladder) = FOUNDATIONS & STRUCTURE

Understanding the TCM Correspondences

5 Elements	WOOD	FIRE	EARTH	METAL	WATER
COLOUR	Green	Red	Yellow	White	Black
SEASONS	Spring	Summer	Late Summer	Autumn	Winter
ENVIRONMENT	Wind	Heat	Damp	Dry	Cold
ZANG	Liver	Heart	Spleen	Lung	Kidney
FU	Gallbladder	Small Intestine	Stomach	Large Intestine	Bladder
DIRECTIONS	East	South	Middle	West	North
TASTES	Sour	Bitter	Sweet	Pungent	Salty
SENSE ORGANS	Eye	Tongue	Mouth	Nose	Ear
TISSUES	Muscle & Tendon	Blood Vessels	Flesh & Limbs	Skin & Hair	Bone
EMOTIONS	Anger	Joy	Worry	Grief	Fear

I find a useful way to understand the Correspondences comes from looking at Chinese culture as historically being agrarian and rural – the bulk of the population were farmers living on the land and they lived in relationship to the cycles of the seasons in nature.

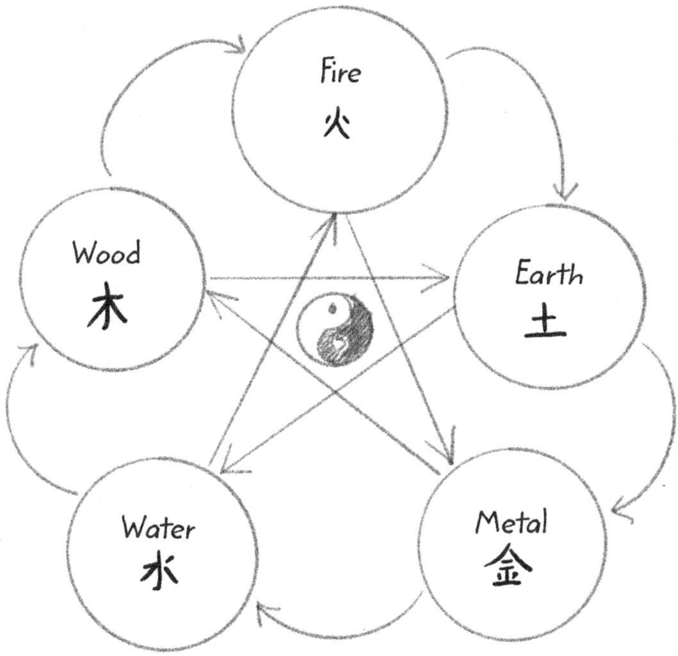

Five Elements Diagram

This gives us:

The cycle of the seasons begins with Spring. This is the time of rebirth of nature after winter. Seeds germinate and sprout, and plants grow vigorously. This is the theme of Spring. Green is the colour of all the lush plant growth and Wood is produced by the growing plants. This is the time of strong Winds and unstable weather – which can give people allergies and make them cranky (Anger).

The Liver and liverish people are vulnerable to disturbance and illness in Spring.

Next comes Summer. Summer is hot and is a time of strong mature Growth of the crops. The Heat of Summer can be associated with Fires (including bushfires) – the colour of Fire is Red.

Pleasant Summer weather fills us with Joy – but to excess this can become Mania.

The Fire Organs (and Heart people) can be thrown out of balance in the Hot Summer.

Then we get to Late Summer. This is the time when the crops reach Maturation and are ready for first harvest. The colour of mature wheat and other crops is gold, Yellow or Orange. This is the time of harvesting the crops and collecting plants.

In this way the Earth nourishes us as plants are Transformed into food for us to eat.

However, if the crops get soaked by rain at harvest or are stored in damp conditions they spoil. Therefore, Dampness can disturb the Earth element and Spleen people.

A great theme of this time is digestion and nourishment – nourishment physically (digestive and hormonal) and mentally. And if a person cannot digest their experiences, they develop repetitive thinking and Obsession. On the other hand, a well-balanced person who digests and integrates all they experience in life is calm and Meditative – almost like a cow chewing her cud.

Next comes Autumn. A time of winds which dry out leaves on the trees and the crops. This Drying process turns things White. Leaves fall from the trees. This is the time of Air in motion - in China this was seen as Metal in its gaseous form = vapour, or perhaps as the fumes rising up from the blacksmith's work as he repairs the metal ploughs and mends things for the upcoming winter. This is also the time of the second or last harvest – hence Reaping.

This focus on Air gives us a relationship to the Respiratory

System. And people who breathe out a lot (sighing) are prone to Melancholy. The Metal element and Lung people are prone to sickness in Autumn.

Finally, we come to Winter. This is the time of death and decay. The crops have withered and turned Black. Everything shrinks back to its fundamental structure or bony skeleton (Bones). People rely on the food and produce they have Stored for the long dark times of Winter. This is also a time of cold and heavy rains - Water is abundant. The Water element and Kidney people tend to get chilled and sick in Winter – coughs, colds, back pain, and arthritis in the joints, are all common. This can lead to a sense of insecurity or Fear about health. And Kidney people can pass water (urine) a lot – bladder urging is associated with Fear – such as just before exams.

CHAPTER 18

Simple Practical TCM

The most common "TCM Syndromes" seen in medical practice in Australia

Liverish

Is the most frequent syndrome – symptoms and signs include anger, irritability, depression, jealousy, headaches, migraines, muscles aches and pains, bad taste in mouth on waking, skin rashes such as eczema, heartburn, allergies, hayfever, and painful periods in women.

"Advanced Liver Syndrome" can include severe inflammatory diseases such as rheumatoid arthritis, Crohn's disease, multiple sclerosis, and also advanced cardiovascular disease (vasculopathy).

In essence the mind and body are irritable.

In TCM this is seen in the syndromes:

> **Ascending Liver Fire (Yang)** – red face, red eyes, migraine, throbbing tension headaches, tinnitus, dizziness, insomnia, high blood pressure, hot flushes, gastro-oesophageal reflux,

flaring anger, constant bitter taste in mouth, red tongue. Often due to prolonged stress, unhealthy diet or alcohol/drug abuse. Treat with LR3, LR2, BL18, GB20.

Deficient Liver Yin – chronic fatigue, chronic liver disease, red face, red tongue. Treat with LR3, LR2, BL18, SP6, KI3, BL23.

Stagnant Liver Qi – pain and tenderness along the Liver / Gallbladder meridians (such as temporal or occipito-frontal headaches, TMJ pain, shoulder pain, sciatica, hip and knee pain), chronic tension (both physically and mentally), depression, frustration, irritability, sensation of distension/ bloating in abdomen or chest. Treat with The Four Gates (bilateral LI4 and LR3)

Spleen Deficiency

Is the next most common – symptoms and signs include fatigue, heaviness, oedema, obesity, heavy periods, hot flushes.

In fact, heaviness is a keynote.

In TCM this is seen as:

Spleen Qi Deficiency – fatigue, oedema, poor digestion, irritable bowel syndrome, chronic diarrhoea, prolapse, heavy periods, tongue is pale and puffy with tooth indented edges and a white coat. Treat with SP6, SP3, ST36, CV12, LR3, BL20.

Spleen Yang deficiency – as above plus cold extremities and feeling chilled. Treat with points as for Spleen Qi Deficiency PLUS CV3, CV6, CV4 with Moxa.

Kidney Deficiency

Symptoms and signs include anxiety, fears, phobias, wandering aches, coldness in kidney area (loins), weak knees, urinary frequency, "neurasthenia" (nervous weakness).

The whole mind and body seem weak and wobbly.

In TCM this is seen as four syndromes:

Kidney Qi Deficiency with back pain, poor memory, impotence, urinary dribbling and incontinence, hair loss, poor hearing, dizziness, pale puffy tongue and white coat. Treat with KI3, SP6, ST36, CV4, CV6, BL23, GV4.

Kidney Yang Deficiency – as for Kidney Qi Deficiency with cold extremities and feeling chilled. Treat as for Kidney Qi Deficiency PLUS KI7, LU9, LI11, GB25, moxa.

Generalised Qi Deficiency – all organ function is slow and deficient with slow speech, slow thinking, exhaustion, with pale face and pale tongue. Treat with ST36, SP6, CV6, CV4, BL20, alarm and associated points of the involved organs.

Deficiency of Jing – the most severe state with debility, great weakness, premature aging, cognitive decline, brittle bones. Treat with herbs, Qigong, and meditation.

Other less common syndromes seen in Western medical practice include:

Heart Excess – overly exuberant, hypomania, talks too much and too quickly, hysteria.

Heart Deficiency– apathy, lack of joy, fatigue, palpitations.

Lung Deficiency – chronic lung disease, depression (melancholia).

CHAPTER 19

Pulse And Tongue Diagnosis – My Take On This

My approach to pulse and tongue diagnosis follows that of Anton Jayasuriya and Geoff Greenbaum.

I find that tongue and pulse diagnosis can be useful sources of information to confirm patterns of disease first picked up by a comprehensive history, both western medical and TCM.

However, I would never rely on just the findings of tongue or pulse diagnosis to decide on a course of action.

All the information from history, tongue and pulses, and western medical examination need to be combined together to make a complete diagnosis and formulate a treatment plan.

Pulse Diagnosis

I find the pulses can give a useful indicator of the person's current state, both physically and psychologically.

As such the pulses can change rapidly, even on an hourly basis.

Pulse diagnosis is performed by the doctor and patient sitting relaxed with arms well supported, the doctor seated in front of the patient.

The doctor places his/her 3rd fingers over the patient's radial pulses at the level of the radial styloid process.

Then the doctor places his/her 2nd and 4th fingers on either side of the 3rd fingers.

Firstly, feel for the overall strength and quality of the pulses.

Then palpate each pulse position lightly at first, then deeply so as to almost occlude the pulse.

Each pulse position corresponds to an element in TCM.

For example, the middle pulse on the patient's left hand corresponds to the wood element = liver / gallbladder.

The superficial pulse position corresponds to the hollow Yang organ of that element, while the deep pulse indicates the state of the related solid Yin organ.

This will then give you a good assessment of the pulses and any indicated patterns of disturbance.

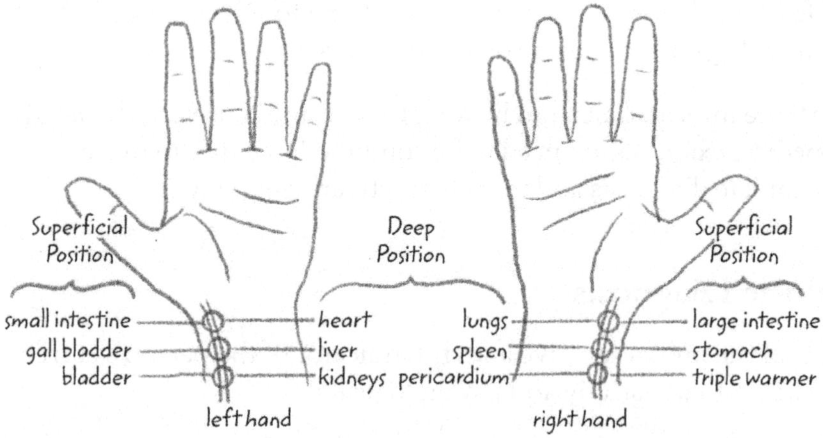

Pulse Diagnosis

Note that there are different views about the nature of the most proximal pulses. Some people see these as BL/KI in the patient's left hand, and TE/PC for the right hand, whereas others (myself included) see these proximal pulses as BL/KI in both hands.

The patterns I look for are:

Overall strength of pulses

Overall rate of the pulse – for example:

Rapid pulses = heat in TCM terms

Slow = cold

Overall quality of pulses – for example:

Spiky = liverish /acute pain / general toxicity

Slippery = spleen

Heavy = pregnant

Hollow / collapsing = "empty spleen pulse"

Generalised very weak pulses or cannot be felt at all = kidney deficiency

Specific pulse positions (as per the diagram), whether excess or deficient in each position

You can then put all this information together to see whether it fits a recognised pattern of organ disturbance, a synthesis of data indicating an overall picture.

Pulse diagnosis is very much an art which takes years to learn well.

It is usually best to feel a lot of pulses in the company of an expert who can guide you in what to find.

Geoff Greenbaum used to say that a student needs to feel at least 100 pulses supervised by a competent pulse diagnostician, and then the student can become competent in the art.

Having said that, I have found that many doctors can learn to pick up the key aspects of pulse diagnosis quite quickly and with a reasonable degree of inter-practitioner agreement, when well taught.

Tongue Diagnosis

The tongue tends to indicate the state of the person's metabolism over a longer period of time – usually weeks to months.

The tongue body gives an indicator of the basic constitution, while the tongue coating tends to show disturbances in metabolism and function.

Changes in the shape or colour of the tongue body and in any tongue coating relate to the part of the tongue they occur on, and correspond with a particular organ.

Before examining the tongue, it is always important to check whether the person is a smoker.

Smoking routinely causes a thick dirty coat on the tongue. This may not be of any real importance (apart from fooling the unwary observer), or it may in fact indicate the significant disturbance that smoking is causing to the person's body. You have to decide which in each individual case.

I am here sharing the information I have gained from my teachers Geoff Greenbaum and Anton Jayasuriya, and which I have found useful in clinical practice.

I acknowledge that classical TCM has some different views about tongue diagnosis.

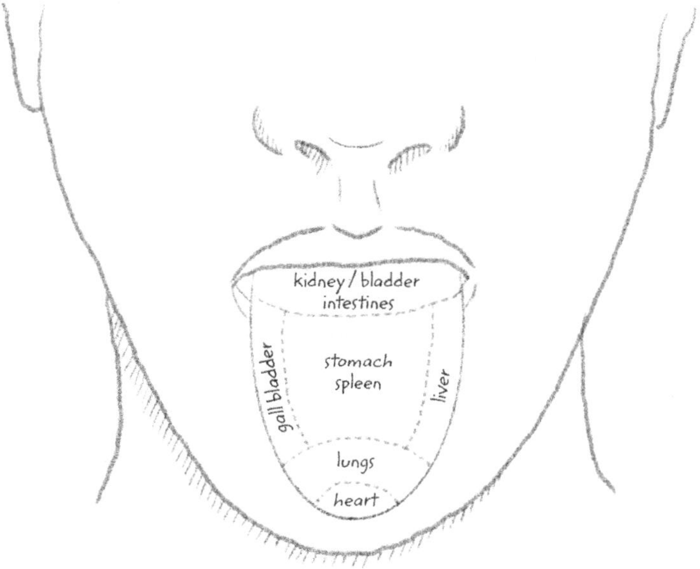

Tongue Diagnosis

A normal tongue is pink, well-shaped, and has either a clear coating or a very thin slightly hazy white coat.

The colour and thickness of any coating on the tongue indicate the depth and chronicity of the disease condition.

Acute superficial disturbance = White thin coat

↓

Disturbance becoming chronic = Creamy or yellowish coat on the tongue

↓

Deep chronic ingrained disease = Thick dark coat on all or key parts of the tongue, and often

with relevant changes in the tongue shape

In the tongue chart above, the tongue edges are usually ascribed to both liver and gall bladder together.

Some typical changes to look for:

Blue or purple colouring of the tongue edges (including blueish veins in this area) suggest the person is Liverish (often stagnant Liver Qi in TCM terms). In advanced stages the whole tongue body may become purplish.

Swelling of the tongue edges suggests Spleen abnormality – as does a generally puffy tongue.

Tooth indented edges of the tongue suggest Spleen or Kidney deficiency – more likely to be Kidney if the tongue is not swollen.

The tooth indentation can also suggest a general Yin state due to Yang deficiency.

A greasy white or cream coating on the tongue suggests mucus from Spleen Dampness. This is often diagnosed medically as oral thrush, but may well not be. It is often simply Spleen Dampness, a tongue change reflecting the general state of the body and not a specific disease in itself. Of course, this state of dampness is perfect for candida to multiply, so the dampness / excess mucus and the candiasis can interact.

A red tip to the tongue suggests Heart excess or Acute Excess Heat – someone who is too revved-up.

Deep central cracks in the body of the tongue suggest Chronic Excess Heat. I liken this to what happens when you are sitting in your car with the engine turned on, foot flat to the floor on the accelerator pedal, but the other foot is on the brake pedal at the same time. The engine starts to overheat and ultimately will break down. A person who is running with Chronic Excess Heat will also break down sooner or later.

TCM sees this deep central grove as Stomach Yin Deficiency.

Multiple cracks all over the tongue suggest chronic allergies. This is more pronounced if there are also pealing areas of the tongue – the so-called "geographic tongue". It is a state of advanced body stress (chronic excess heat) with multiple allergies.

A thin tongue suggests a generally deficient state.

Overly strong tongue protrusion suggests a Yang state of general excess.

A timid tongue protrusion, especially with trembling of the tongue, suggests a general deficient or Yin state.

A thin white coat suggests Lung Excess – for example in acute eczema, acute asthma, or an acute upper respiratory tract infection (the common cold).

Dark tongue coating towards the rear of the tongue suggests disturbance of the intestines or of the Kidney Qi.

Dark blotches on the tongue can be due to parasites or to Stagnant Blood in TCM terms.

A generally pale tongue suggests a generally deficient state.

A generally reddened tongue suggests a state of excess, especially excess heat.

CHAPTER 20

Cultivating And Projecting Your Qi

Cultivate your own Qi

This involves a combination of healthy lifestyle, good nutrition, good restful sleep, regular relaxation and stillness, living in a minimally polluted healthy environment, and cultivating a positive peaceful state of mind. Nature has wonderful effects.

Practise Qigong and meditation

This ancient Chinese practice is a great way to clear the acupuncture meridians and build your Qi. Over time you can directly experience the energy of the organs and channels in both health and dis-ease / disease.

Project Qi during the treatment

There are various ways to do this, whether by Qigong or other approaches such as reiki, "blessing the patient", or simply wishing them well as you perform the acupuncture.

Best learned from a practitioner who has mastered this art.

CHAPTER 21

From My Teachers

Dr. Geoff Greenbaum

Dr. Geoffrey Greenbaum was an experienced general practitioner in Melbourne, and was involved with medical education at the Royal Australian College of General Practitioners for many years.

He became very keen to find out more about acupuncture, and in 1974 went to Hong Kong to study with a cardio-thoracic surgeon Dr. Huang who was also an expert acupuncturist.

Over time Geoff further learnt from study trips to China, visits to Dr. Felix Mann in London, Dr. Anton Jayasuriya in Sri Lanka, and Prof. Johannes Bischko in Vienna.

Geoff then became a full-time medical acupuncturist and after Dr. John Woodley retired in the late 1970's from running the acupuncture research clinic he had set up at Preston And Northcote Community Hospital (PANCH), Geoff subsequently ran that acupuncture clinic at PANCH and later The Northern Hospital, Epping, until he retired in 2002.

Geoff set up excellent acupuncture training courses for doctors firstly with the Royal Australian College of General Practitioners, then at PANCH, and finally he created the Graduate Diploma of Medical Acupuncture which ran at Monash University from the mid-1990's until 2013.

Key Teachings From Dr. Geoff Greenbaum:

Geoff was always keen to apply the scientific method to acupuncture – to observe what actually happened, to then reason from that observation and to test ideas against reality. He was not bound by old theories. Instead, Geoff was interested in what was actually seen to work in his patients.

Acupuncture works mainly via HOMOEOSTASIS. Therefore, there is no need to specifically "sedate" or "tonify" acupuncture points during treatment. The simple act of stimulating the point with the needle or laser will set off a self-correcting process for that meridian / organ.

The Art of Good Acupuncture is being able to find Reactive Points on the patient's body – and then knowing which of these reactive points to actually treat on the given day of treatment.

This is a parallel to Dr. Felix Mann's teaching that "acupuncture points" do not exist as such. Instead, there are regions of sensitisation with specific responses to acupuncture stimulation, which occur somewhere near to classic acupuncture points, but are in fact quite variable as to both location and size. These places for acupuncture stimulation are not rigid or "set in stone" as specific locations on a map. Instead use the acupuncture point descriptions to get you into the general body region and then use your fingers to palpate (and sometimes your eyes to look for local tissue change, such as local swelling, blood vessel abnormalities, tissue thickening, or skin crusting) and find the actual Reactive Point which you will then treat.

A Tranquillising Sequence is always worth a try – especially if there is NOT a good response to the treatment program. These "tranquillising points" are so named because they have a recognised effect on the emotions to calm, sedate and balance the person's mood state.

This can include use of some or all of the recognised "tranquillising points" – GV15, GV20, LI4, PC6, HT7 +/- Ear Shenmen or HT3.

Sishencong and Yintang (which has a powerful effect on the frontal lobes, limbic system and hypothalamus) may also be useful.

In "stuck cases" try:

Tranquillising Sequence

"Inner Gate" (Neiguan) and "Outer Gate" (Weiguan) together (PC6 + TE5) to rebalance the superficial and deep energy flow

KI27 – end point of the Kidney meridian – powerfully enhancing of Essential Kidney Qi

SP21 – "Associated Point of all points"

Unexpected curtailing of response – In previously good responders who now unexpectedly stop responding well, or who now only repeatedly get response lasting only a few days, consider the development of underlying pathology:

Occult neoplasm

Major psycho-pathology or socio-cultural problems

Major inflammatory, infective or auto-immune disease

Geoff often used Dr. Felix Mann's "Periosteal Points" with good benefit.

No need to use a needle to actually "peck" these points down to the periosteum – just stimulate them as per normal acupuncture points

These Periosteal Points include:

Tender points around the margin of any joint

Tender points at teno-periosteal junctions

Lateral and Medial Epicondyle of the elbow – for tennis elbow and golfer's elbow respectively

Coracoid Process medial to the head of the humerus (near LU1) – for shoulder / arm pain

Cervical Transverse Processes in the neck – for neck / arm pain and headaches. Note: If needling you must approach posteriorly, to avoid puncturing the vertebral artery (a risk with an anterior approach)

Sacro-Iliac Joint (SIJ) – for back and hip pain

ASIS – anterior superior iliac spine for groin and anterior hip pain

Iliac Crest – posteriorly for back pain

Greater Trochanter of the femoral head – for hip pain

Medial Condyle of the tibia (superior to SP9) – for knee pain

Anterior Tip of Calcaneus underneath the heel – for plantar fasciitis and "heel spur"

"Felix Mann's BL62" – 1 cun below the tip of the lateral malleolus of the ankle on the calcaneal ridge (below classical BL62). If tender, this can be a better point for local ankle pain, distal point for neck / shoulder pain, and as the "unofficial influential point" for problems of the nervous system, both peripheral and central

Geoff Greenbaum's and Anton Jayasurija's **"Classic Point Sequences":**

Influential Points

BL11 – bone, cartilage, joints

GB34 / LR3 – muscles, tendons

LU9 – blood vessels, circulatory system

CV17 – respiratory system, Qi

CV12 – hollow organs, Fu

LR13 – solid organs, Zang

BL17 – blood

GB39 – marrow

Command Point

GV26 – collapse, resuscitation

Area Of Influence Points

LI4 - face

LU7 – side of neck

PC6 – chest & epigastrium

ST36 – abdomen

SP6 – pelvis & pelvic organs & inner legs

BL40 – back & back of legs

Alarm and Associated Points – Back Shu and Mu Front Points

Points on the front of the body (Alarm / Mu points) and on the back of the body (Associated / Shu points) along the Bladder meridian, which have a powerful effect on the relevant organ.

Some people suggest that Mu points are used in acute illness and Shu points on the back are used in chronic illness. However, Geoff used these points interchangeably, and often in pairs. He would often feel for the most reactive point, to decide whether to use the Mu Front or Back Shu point.

Some key examples include:

Lung: LU1 / BL13

Heart: CV14 / BL15

Liver: LR14 / BL18

Gall Bladder: GB24 / BL19

Spleen: LR13 / BL20

Kidney: GB25 / BL23

Large Intestine: ST25 / BL25

Bladder: CV3 / BL28

Confluent Points

Pairs of points with widespread effect on extensive regions of the body

Eg SI3 + BL62 – for all spine, especially neck

Great Points

These are points which have a very powerful effect on many functions, and are often used in treatment

LI4, ST36, SP6

Felix Mann would add LR3 to this list as his favourite point

Physiological Points – points with recognised physiological effects:

Analgesic - LI4, ST44

Anti-inflammatory - GV14, LI4, LI11, ST36, SP6

Immune Enhancing - GV14, LI4, LI11, ST36, SP6

Anti-allergy - SP10

Tranquillising - GV15, GV20, LI4, PC6, HT7, (HT3)

Tonifying for low vitality - GV14, LI4, ST36, SP6, (CV6)

Homoeostatic – LI4, LI11, ST36, SP6

Periosteal Points – bony tender points as per Felix Mann

Points with Specific Effects – such as:

ST38 for frozen shoulder

Tim-Mee point for smoking addiction

This is a new point found on the back of the wrist as a very tender lump approximately 1 cun from LU7. It is close to TE5.

Spheno-Palatine Ganglion on the face

Geoff Greenbaum did significant pioneering hospital work with:

Acupuncture Anaesthesia for open cholecystectomy.

This was performed successfully at St. George's Hospital in Kew, Melbourne, from 1977 onwards. One such successful procedure was filmed.

Based on these experiences, Geoff's comments were that Acupuncture Anaesthesia was successful but time consuming.

In the Australian hospital environment Acupuncture Anaesthesia is not very useful, given that medical labour is expensive whereas the medications for chemical anaesthesia are cheap.

However, in China the reverse is true – labour is inexpensive but the anaesthetic medications are costly. Hence this is a useful technique in China.

In China sometimes the Acupuncture Anaesthesia needs to be supplemented by light sedation or local anaesthesia.

The bottom line is that Acupuncture Anaesthesia is a useful technique – especially for patients with allergies or problematic side effects to the anaesthetic medications.

Pilot studies in a hospital setting with a surgeon at PANCH on:

Pre-operative Acupuncture (1 session within 10 days prior to the surgery with Immune Enhancing Points chosen from LI4, GV14, ST36, SP6, LR3) for open cholecystectomy. Results (unpublished) showed that post-operative complications were reduced by 50%, and patients on average were able to be discharged from hospital 1 day sooner. This amounted to a significant cost saving for the hospital.

Healing resistant Varicose Ulcers – after the second skin transplant had broken down. In this 3-month study 2/3 of the enrolled patients had complete healing of the varicose ulcer. The remaining patients all had ulcer healing over the next 6 months. Points used were:

> Points on the meridians crossing the ulcer above and below the ulcer
>
> LU9 (Influential Point of the blood vessels)
>
> Sometimes a "constitutional point" eg LR3 for a "liverish person" or SP6 for someone who was "spleen deficient".
>
> Spray the ulcer and the surrounding tissue margin with laser. The laser used was the 1.5mW HeNe 632.8nm red light Silberbauer laser applied at 1 square cm per minute.

These unpublished pilot studies obviously need to be repeated on a much larger scale. Nevertheless, they indicate interesting possibilities with acupuncture.

Ear Acupuncture:

Ear points are often very useful. Use ear acupuncture early in treatment if there are not good responses to body points (after the first 2 to 4 treatment if slow response to body points).

Ear points have a powerful effect but are NOT likely to cause an aggravation.

Sometimes there may be a few days delay in response to treatment with ear points – but this does not always apply. There can on occasion be immediate powerful positive response to a well-chosen ear point.

Midline Body Points:

These are LESS likely to cause aggravations than distal limb points but can still be potent yet gentle.

Order Of Potency of Acupuncture Points – from most potent to least:

Distal Body Points tend to have powerful effects, but can easily aggravate a sensitive patient

Ear Points – usually do NOT cause aggravations

Midline Body Points are generally much less potent in effect

For a Sensitive Delicate Patient, to minimise the chance of aggravation, use:

Ear Points

Midline Body Points (GV or CV meridian – such as GV20 or GV15)

Geoff Greenbaum's simplified approach to TCM:

I have found this approach to work very well.

Firstly, if possible, identify the Key Organ Disturbance.

An organ disturbance may not always be present – especially in acute cases or in simple localised musculo-skeletal problems.

The Key Organ Disturbances in order of frequency (most to least common) as seen in Western medical practice:

Liver – the "liverish person". Often in TCM would be diagnosed as "stagnant liver Qi" or as "ascending liver fire"

Spleen – often in TCM this is "Spleen Qi Deficiency"or "Spleen Dampness"

Kidney – often in TCM this is Kidney Qi Deficiency, but also may be Yin or Yang Deficiency

Lung – usually Qi Deficiency

Heart – Qi Deficiency or Excess

Secondly, once identified treat the Key Organ Disturbance with acupuncture on the basis that acupuncture primarily works by Homoeostasis – hence it does not matter if the organ / meridian is "excess" or deficient".

All you need to do is to use a key point on the meridian for the organ disturbance, and then the organ and meridian function will automatically rebalance.

Usually this is via the Yuan Source Point of the meridian – although sometimes you might use the He Sea Point or another Great Point on the meridian.

Typical Examples:

LR3 for a "liverish" person

SP6 for someone with "spleen deficiency"

KI3 for a person with "kidney deficiency"

In summary, there is usually no need to go into the details of diagnosing specific organ disturbances as done in TCM.

But you do need these detailed TCM diagnoses to prescribe Chinese herbs.

For acupuncture, an understanding of the fundamentals of TCM is important, especially as it applies to the sort of patients in your individual practice (for example my practice is dominated by Anglo-Saxons and Celts, with a fair sprinkling of people of Mediterranean origin, and a few from the Indian subcontinent).

Overall, in chronic conditions (which is by far the bulk of my practice) use a powerful point on the meridian relating to the organ disturbance.

This is usually the Yuan Source point or sometimes the He Sea point on that meridian.

Remember that acupuncture is understood to work primarily by inducing homoeostasis (according to Felix Mann, Geoff Greenbaum and Anton Jayasuriya), and so any powerful point on the relevant meridian will be able to induce this effect, especially if this point has good autonomic innervation.

Given that "liverish" problems are the most common in my practice, I use LR3 a lot. This is followed by SP6 for the "spleen deficient" patients, and then KI3 for the "kidney deficiency" patients.

Dr. Felix Mann

I indirectly learned from Dr. Mann through the teaching of Dr. Geoff Greenbaum, who was strongly influenced by Dr. Mann.

Dr. Felix Mann was a gifted general practitioner in London, England.

He became interested in the possibilities of acupuncture shortly after it became known in the Western world.

Dr. Mann was one of the first people to translate some of the ancient Chinese texts into English in the 1960's.

He also carried out some of the early research into how acupuncture might work.

His demonstration of "viscero-somatic" and "somato-visceral" reflexes is still important today.

> In experimental work with rats, Dr. Mann noticed that stimulation to a specific point just below the joint of the rat's hindleg (below the "knee" – equivalent to the acupoint Stomach 36), would produce reflex contractions of the large intestine. This was in accordance with the teachings of TCM where ST36 is known as the "Area Of Influence Point" for the abdomen (and thus the large intestine). This was called a Somato-Visceral Reflex.
>
> In addition, Dr. Mann found that if a surgical nick was applied to the rat's large intestine, it would start spontaneously chewing at the area just below its knee – at ST36. This was called the Viscero-Somatic Reflex.
>
> Dr. Mann then showed that these reflex responses were abolished if the rat's spinal cord was cut through (transected).
>
> This was good early work to show that the spinal cord and related nerve arcs were important in acupuncture effects.

Dr. Mann was a great observer and over time took a great interest in what actually works in the medical practice of acupuncture. Through this work he adapted the traditional Chinese rules of how to perform acupuncture to meet the very significant differences of Anglo-Celtic westerners.

Dr. Mann was a gifted teacher and lectured in Australia in 1976, exposing a number of medical doctors to his carefully thought-through ideas about acupuncture.

Dr. Mann also noticed that the rigidity of some of the teaching of Traditional Chinese Medicine was overdone, and in time he came to question many of these teachings. In his later years he came up with a more simplified view of acupuncture, and he went so far as to state that there was no such thing as an acupuncture point. (I believe he was saying this in relationship to the fixed "geographical" descriptions of acupoints in the textbooks. Instead, he taught that you must examine the individual patient and find their individual specific regions of tissue reactivity).

Dr. Mann's final thoughts are expressed in his brilliant iconoclastic book "Re-inventing Acupuncture", especially the Second Edition.

So, to some key ideas from Dr. Felix Mann:

In "white Caucasians" many illnesses have a "Liverish basis".

This relates to a pattern of illness recognised in both TCM and European folk medicine as aches and pains, occipito-frontal headaches, migraines, allergies including eczema, hayfever and asthma, dyspepsia and reflux, tendency to arthritis and inflammation, changed liver metabolism of alcohol, drugs and various medications (either "one pot screamers" or "can drink like a fish"), irritability, anger, frustration, and resentment.

In advanced stages of the liver syndrome, we get chronic inflammatory and auto-immune diseases such as multiple sclerosis, rheumatoid arthritis, lupus (SLE), inflammatory bowel disease (such as Crohn's Disease), and advanced vasculopathy such as recurrent angina, heart attacks, strokes, or arterial blockage in the legs.

These patterns are traditionally ascribed to dysfunction of liver metabolism, although evidence about this is unclear from the Western medicine point of view.

Therefore, LR3 is often useful in many patients – and may be the key point or even only point of the treatment.

LR3 is the Yuan Source point for the Liver channel.

If LR3 is too strong and might, or actually does, aggravate the patient's condition, the HeSea point of the Liver channel can be used instead – LR8.

In chronic conditions we tend to use the points on the involved meridian which store the most energy and therefore the most powerful effects. These are:

> **The Yuan Source Point** – usually around the ankle or wrist. "The place where the Qi is deepest" where the Original Qi of the organ is housed.
>
> **The HeSea Point** – usually at the knee or elbow. "The place where the Qi flows most broadly".

People of Chinese or Indian/Pakistani/Sri Lankan origin are known to be hyper-sensitive to stimulation of LR3. They may have an excessive vagal response and so drop their blood pressure or even collapse. (If this occurs, all that is needed is to lie the patient down and rest them until recovered.)

Therefore, use LR3 with great care in people of Chinese or Indian genetics, or don't use it at all - as recommended by Prof. Dr. Sir Anton Jayasuriya.

Felix Mann reminds us of the ancient maxim from the old Chinese texts "The Master Acupuncturist uses only one needle."

There is great wisdom in this.

There is often just one point which is the key to treatment, and this can be all that is needed.

Too often far too many points are used – and this can detract from the effectiveness of the treatment.

At the very least these extra points add nothing to the treatment, but too often they inhibit the effectiveness of the treatment, and may even cause aggravations or totally miss the patient's "window of responsiveness" and therefore have no benefit at all.

Having said that, there is never a hard and fast in rule in acupuncture, because we humans are so varied as individuals. So, there will be some patients who do need many points treated – but it is usually wise to work up to this gradually over time.

A great rule of thumb is "If in doubt use one point only – especially at the beginning of the treatment program".

Stimulating anywhere in the same body region will produce some therapeutic acupuncture effect.

Depending on the sensitivity of the patient, this responsive body region may vary from the same neurological segment (eg dermatome), through the same limb, to the same ipsilateral body half, and even to the whole body.

Specific treatment of the actual exact reactive acupuncture point will have a better therapeutic effect. But stimulating the relevant reactive region of the body will still have some good benefit.

Do not forget about this generalised non-specific response to needling. It all too often confounds attempts to use "control treatment" in scientific studies of acupuncture, and renders such "sham acupuncture" as rubbish for a placebo control. You end up comparing very good acupuncture with basic acupuncture – both are treatments with positive results.

In studies, to see a genuine statistical difference between "true acupuncture" and "sham acupuncture" treatment on areas on the body away from points classically described in the texts, very large numbers of patients are needed in the two groups – typically numbering in the thousands.

Scientific thinking is just starting to catch up with this understanding, but there is still a long way to go before the scientific community in general understands that it is virtually impossible to carry out valid placebo-controlled studies in acupuncture.

Acupuncture really needs different styles of analysis compared to the double-blind placebo-controlled studies which are appropriate for study of pharmaceutical drugs.

Felix Mann described the concept of Strong Responders.

This applies to patients who get a far greater therapeutic response than expected, from a given treatment. These patients usually only require a few points to get maximum benefit – often only one point with minimal or no stimulation.

Very gentle forms of acupuncture are preferred for these patients – such as ear acupuncture, Japanese acupuncture (a quick "in and out" superficial insertion of a very fine needle just through the skin, and no deeper), or laser acupuncture.

Felix Mann thought that about 20% of patients belonged to this group. But in his later years he found that up to 40% of his patients were Strong Responders. He theorised this may be due to his treatment techniques getting better, or to attracting more of such patients through word mouth, or perhaps because he expected most of his patients to be Strong Responders and so this expectation maximised the responsiveness of all his patients – as a very strong placebo effect.

I have noticed that "birds of a feather flock together".

Once you get good results with some Strong Responder patients, they start to send all their friends and family to you – and fortunately they are usually Strong Responders too. The reverse also applies – you can get a string of very average responders coming to you once one or several such mediocre responders start sending people to you.

There is a natural tendency for people to associate with others of a similar nature.

And acupuncture response appears to be genetic – it runs in families.

I would add that children are almost always Strong Responders.

And long-term practitioners of meditation, yoga, tai chi, or qigong are also virtually universally Strong Responders.

Subsequently the concept of *Hyper-Reactors* was developed.

This is the observation that some patients, who might or might not have originally been Strong Responders, through the challenges of life have become very depleted and so tend to easily aggravate from any form of treatment, but often get no benefit from the treatment.

These people too often have fallen foul of over-aggressive Western medical treatment and have paid the price. They get aggravations from just about anything and are very hard to help.

You can on occasion do some good for these Hyper-Reactors by avoiding local points and use just one or two general points.

These general points may just focus on the key disturbing process, such as severely depleted vitality, major stress effects, or severe immune dysfunction.

Over time a single point might then be added in for specific pain problems, but never use a local point in the area of pain – unless the patient's general condition has improved greatly, and they are in essence no longer a "hyper-reactor".

This is a reason why our hospital acupuncture clinic was popular with medical specialists and surgeons at PANCH and later at The Northern Hospital. We were able to help at least 50% of their "failures" and provide genuine improvement in quality of life for these patients. These were obviously people who had become Hyper-Reactors from problems relating to their illnesses, and from the intensive treatments they had received at the hospital. Hence our clinic was well supported by both the specialists and also, more importantly, by the hospital patients.

Dr. Anton Jayasuriya

Anton was Professor of Rheumatology and Chief Acupuncturist at Colombo South General Hospital, Kalubowila, Sri Lanka.

He was trained as an acupuncturist in China, and during his lifetime treated over 250,000 patients at the hospital in Sri Lanka.

He was a gifted teacher and speaker, with a great understanding of Traditional Chinese Medicine. He travelled the world and taught over 6,000 acupuncturists from a range of countries.

He was also something of a non-conformist and liked to do things his own way. Yet his charm and charisma carried all before him.

A loveable rogue indeed.

Some of Anton's teachings:

As an aid to remember the Six Area Of Influence Points.

These are the acupuncture points which relate to specific body regions – if you like to areas of geography on the body.

Anton used the imagery of a cat washing itself:

> First the cat licks its paw then rubs this over its face. This gives LI4 as Area Of Influence Point (AOIP) for the face.
>
> Next the cat licks the side of its wrist then washes its neck with its paw. This gives LU7 as the AOIP for the side of the neck.
>
> The cat then licks the front of its wrist then rubs its chest. This gives PC6 as the AOIP for the chest and upper stomach.
>
> Next the cat licks its knee then straightens up, rubbing its paw over its belly. This gives ST36 as the AOIP for the abdomen.
>
> Then the cat licks its shin then pulls its paws up over the pelvic area. This gives SP6 as the AOIP for the pelvis and pelvic organs.

> Finally, the cat licks the back of its knee and stretches out, drawing its paw up across its back. This gives BL40 as the AOIP for the back.

To remember the sides of the body corresponding with Yin and Yang. The Yin side of the body (feminine energy) is right, so Anton's maxim was "The woman is always in the right."

This principle is very useful if you don't want to use Distal Points bilaterally – if you want to keep the points to a minimum in a sensitive patient, yet get maximum benefit from the input.

This means that for best effect use a Yang point on the Yang side of the body (left side), and a Yin point on the Yin side of the body (right).

For example, if you want to use the combination of ST36, SP6 and LR3 with minimum input but maximum effect, treat ST36 on the left leg, and SP6 and LR3 on the right leg.

Anton quoted the TCM Husband And Wife Law – "For true harmony the husband should dominate the wife, a little."

I know that this is not politically correct these days (so please don't shoot me), but it does reflect a reality of energy balance, particularly as seen in the pulses.

In other words, the husband (ie. the person with the masculine role and energy) should be the leader in the relationship – but not be a dictator. He should be responsive to and caring for his wife, who carries the feminine nourishing Yin energies.

This applies in Pulse Diagnosis - for proper balance the pulses on the patient's left wrist (Yang – masculine side) should be slightly stronger than those on the right (Yin – feminine side).

Another of Anton's sayings was "If the person has a problem in the head (be it headaches or mental/emotional disturbances), then look to the other end of the body (pelvis and pelvic organs) for the cause.

And vice versa."

This covers such areas as emotional problems connecting to sexual abuse, or chronic constipation related to constant worrying.

Anton quoted a wise old saying "The man (person) behind the needle is more important than the needle."

Anton very wisely recognised that the needle is the least important part of the treatment.

Far more significant is the acupuncturist as a healer – consciously interacting with the patient to support the best healing response possible.

Anton had a wealth of experience and understanding which he communicated to his students with these vivid sorts of teachings.

He got to the core of the matter with these pithy statements.

They stay with you for life.

CHAPTER 22

Laser Acupuncture In My Medical Practice

Laser Acupuncture – How To Do It: The Basics

First, purchase a good quality red light laser in the range 1mW – 60mW emitting a continuous beam.

Silberbauer has always been the gold standard for acupuncture lasers, since the time when they produced the first acupuncture laser for Prof. Johannes Bischko in Vienna in the mid-1970's. I currently use an 8mW 658nm red light CL Mini laser with a power reducing tip, delivering 0.06 Joules per point when applied for the standard 15 seconds. I find this very effective for acupuncture treatment.

If you intend to use the laser for "sports medicine" (Laser Therapy / PBMT) then you may wish to purchase a 60 to 100mw laser – as long as the dose can be dialled down appropriately for acupuncture points.

For all lasers above 5mW power, a divergent beam is preferred for safety reasons.

Otherwise for all lasers above 5mW, and for all infra-red lasers (and I do NOT recommend using these, unless for a special reason), suitable eye protection (goggles) must be worn by the patient, and preferably by the practitioner.

Next decide the laser dose to be applied to each acupoint.

The formula is:

Energy Dose (Joules) = Laser Power (Watts) x Time applied (seconds).

In general laser dose per acupoint in a "standard adult" is in the range of 0.03 – 0.20 Joules per point.

However, I do concede that recent scientific research suggests that a laser dose in the order of at least 0.5 Joules per point is required for effective treatment. My own view based on much personal experience is that this may be true for some "slow/ poor responders" and for non-acupuncture trigger points, but generally with the sort of sensitive patients who come to see me a much lower laser dose works very well. In fact, I have found that in many sensitive patients a too high laser dose is counter-productive, with either reduced effectiveness or even treatment aggravations.

I think the important thing is to understand the nature of the patients who typically come to see you, and then tailor your treatment accordingly (including as regards laser dose per point).

I personally prefer a laser dose for adults around 0.05 Joules per point.

For children and infants, titrate the laser dose per point downwards in the same way as you would if prescribing medication. That is, reduce the dosage according to body weight compared to the average adult.

So, if a child is half the size / weight of an adult, then give them half the energy dose per point.

I usually give infants the briefest stimulation possible – typically 1 second per point.

I generally treat Strong Responders and Hyper-Reactors as if they are children.

If such patients are particularly weakened and sensitised, I treat them with 1 point only, for 1 second.

Thirdly, you must be exact about finding the acupuncture point.

Find the centre of the reactive point – the centre of tenderness, tissue oedema / swelling, fibrous change, change in Electrical Skin Resistance, or energy flare (Qi radiating from the point) at the acupuncture point.

Fourthly, when irradiating large areas with the laser:

I use the formula pioneered by Prof. Bischko for his 1.5mW HeNe 632.8nm red light laser: Slowly move the laser over the treatment area at a rate of 1 square cm per minute.

Obviously for higher power lasers you reduce the time of application accordingly.

For example, with a laser in the region of 5–6mW (roughly 3 times the power of Bischko's HeNe laser) you would apply this laser to the treatment area at a rate of 1 square cm per 20 seconds.

Subtle Approaches I use to enhance acupuncture treatment

Cultivate your own Qi.

Practise Qigong and meditation.

Project Qi during the treatment – there are various ways to do this, whether by Qigong or other approaches such as reiki, "blessing the patient", or simply wishing them well as you perform the acupuncture.

Practical Tips

At the first treatment, assume everyone is a Strong Responder until proven otherwise.

Remember to keep your points to the minimum necessary, especially at the first treatment.

As a rule of thumb at the First Treatment avoid local points – use 1 or 2 well-chosen distal points or ear points. Maximum of 3 points. This reduces the risk of significantly aggravating Strong Responders and Hyper Reactors. This particularly applies in Chronic Conditions.

In general, with laser, use 50% more local points and bilateral distal points compared to needle acupuncture.

However, of course modify this according to the patient's unique responsiveness. For example, use only 1 or 2 points in Strong Responders, no matter what.

In Acute Conditions use 1 or 2 local points, sometimes supported a distal point (usually a distal point on the meridian crossing the area of pain/pathology or an Influential Point for the relevant body tissue) can be very effective.

In acute injury or inflammation, direct application of the laser to the involved tissues can be very helpful. This is Laser Therapy, not Laser Acupuncture.

Frequency Of Treatment

In general treat:

> Hyper Acute Conditions daily until settled – eg Acute Locked Back.

Acute Conditions in general treat every 2 –3 days until settled.

With Hyper Acute and Acute Conditions, it may be worthwhile having a "booster treatment" about 1 week after the condition settles.

Chronic Conditions treat every 1 to 4 weeks.

CHAPTER 23

A Final Thumbnail Overview Of Laser Acupuncture

Laser Acupuncture

Introduction to acupuncture

Acupuncture stimulates specific sensitive points on the body. It can be applied with needles, electrical stimulation, acupressure, ultrasound, dry ice or laser. Acupuncture can relieve symptoms and improve function for many conditions.

How Acupuncture Works

Scientific research has found that there are specific nerve endings at acupuncture points, and these can be stimulated so they send signals to the spinal cord and brain to block transmission of pain impulses.

Acupuncture also sends signals to stimulate the brain to produce certain chemicals (neuropeptides) for pain relief, to improve sleep and relieve depression, and to provide anti-inflammatory, anti-allergy, immune-boosting and vitality-boosting effects.

Acupuncture sends signals from the brain back down the spinal cord to rebalance muscle function and reduce muscle spasm. This can help in chronic pain and in recovery from stroke or head injury.

Acupuncture can stimulate the brain to rebalance function of the autonomic nervous system, which controls the function of organs, nerves, and blood vessels.

Acupuncture can also restore distorted pain perceptions in the brain (neuroplasticity).

Acupuncture can have important effects locally and centrally in the brain to reduce neuro-sensitization in chronic pain.

The view of Traditional Chinese Medicine is that illness is due to imbalance of flow of the body's vital energy (Qi – pronounced "chee") in the organs and through the channels of the body (acupuncture meridians). Pain is thought to be due to a build-up of stagnant Qi behind a blockage or "log-jam" in the meridian. The acupuncture points are special responsive sites on the meridian which can unblock or change the flow of Qi energy in that channel.

Proper medical investigation and diagnosis should always be carried out before commencing acupuncture.

Laser Acupuncture

Laser acupuncture was developed in the 1970's at the University of Vienna. There has been a lot of scientific research since then to confirm that it works and is safe. The red-light laser beam penetrates 1–2mm into the body tissues to stimulate special nerve endings at acupuncture points. These nerve endings then trigger off the acupuncture response.

Scientific studies have demonstrated the effectiveness of laser acupuncture. Further research is needed on the details of exactly how laser acupuncture works.

Laser acupuncture is painless and is a very subtle yet effective stimulus to acupuncture points. Laser is preferable to needle acupuncture for children, sensitive people, and where needle acupuncture is too painful or aggravates the person. There is no risk of infection or of damaging organs with the laser – this can be important in settings such as a patient with immune suppression from chemotherapy treatment, in lymphoedema of the arm after breast cancer surgery, or for a person with seriously impaired circulation in a limb.

Red light laser also stimulates tissue healing.

For further information see the websites:

www.medicalacupuncture.org

www.amac.org.au

Risks, Possible Side Effects and Contra-indications to Laser Acupuncture

Scientific research has shown that low power red light lasers (power range 1 to 100mW, wavelength 630 to 660nm, application time 1 to 60 seconds) used in acupuncture do not cause any tissue damage, either in the short or long term. They do not cause burns and are safe for the body. Research to confirm the safety and effectiveness of these acupuncture lasers has been carried out at the University Of Vienna in Austria, and by many scientific institutions since.

Laser acupuncture should NOT be applied:

Directly into the open eye

Over cancer tissue

Over openings in the skull

To the belly of a pregnant woman

Perhaps over electronic implants – pacemakers etc.

On the head in severe unstable epilepsy

Note: Do not use laser for people with severe EMF sensitivity

CHAPTER 24

Conclusion

Laser Acupuncture has been a wonderful part of my life for many years.

Personally, I love light therapy in all its aspects.

Over the years I have seen many superb responses to this treatment approach, and hence I can profoundly recommend it to you.

As a doctor and a healer, I greatly respect and, as much as possible, live by the fundamental medical maxim of "Primum non nocere":

Firstly, do no harm.

And finally, a principle I am a great believer in:

"The art of good medicine is to do as much nothing as possible"

From "The House Of God" by Dr. Samuel Shem

The aim is to provide just the right type of gentle stimulus to the human organism, at the right time, and delivered in such a way that the system can incorporate and then respond positively to the stimulus, with the maximum benefit possible.

And with minimum harm from the treatment.

As such, it is wise to allow plenty of time for Mother Nature to do her work and to find a new (hopefully healthier) balance for the person, after the initial gentle prod is provided by the practitioner.

You the doctor must then provide any further therapeutic prods, if any, with care and good judgement.

Do not prod again until the patient's system has achieved a new state of balance. Then decide whether any further treatment is useful at that time.

It is very much a "hands off" approach.

This is a therapeutic approach that is gentle, respectful, and truly wholistic.

Light Therapy can indeed be seen as the "medicine of the future".

Laser Acupuncture stands as a key element of this new frontier of medicine.

Wishing you great enjoyment in the practise of this subtle art and science of Laser Acupuncture.

Dr. Ralph Ballard

APPENDIX

Western Medical Acupuncture

Case analysis and treatment prescription

Based on the Teachings of Dr. Felix Mann

Prof. Anton Jayasuriya, Dr. Geoff Greenbaum

And with thanks to all my teaching colleagues

Initial Assessment

Firstly, be a medical doctor – take a Medical History, perform a Clinical Examination, and organise any appropriate extra Tests.

Consider whether the patient needs Referral for further care.

Once you have determined that there are no pressing medical problems requiring immediate attention, then consider whether acupuncture is an appropriate treatment modality for the patient.

If so, discuss the possibility of acupuncture with the patient. Discuss treatment technique, and possible benefits and side effects of the acupuncture treatment.

Take the patient through a written Informed Consent process.

THEN with the patient's consent proceed with acupuncture.

Case Analysis

An approach to formulating your Acupuncture Prescription for the day's treatment:

1. What meridians are involved?
   This relates to meridians crossing the area of disturbance.
2. What organs are involved – if any?
3. Any recognised western medical "physiological" processes involved:
   - Pain
   - Inflammation
   - Infection
   - Allergy
   - Anxiety / Depression
   - Fatigue
4. Indications from Tongue and Pulse Diagnosis – if any
5. Local Points:
   - Local Points on involved meridians
   - Extra Points – numbered and unnumbered
   - Ah Shi points
   - Periosteal Points – as per Felix Mann
6. Distal Points:
   - Distal Points on Involved Meridians
   - Influential Points

- Area Of Influence Points
- Command Points
- Alarm and Associated Points

7. Physiological Points – points with recognised physiological effects:

- Analgesic
- Anti-inflammatory
- Immune Enhancing
- Anti-allergy
- Tranquillising
- Tonifying for low vitality
- Homoeostatic

8. Points by TCM:

- Points from TCM Laws and by TCM Diagnosis:
- Five Element points
- Luo Connecting points
- Mother-Son points
- Horary Points, etc.
- Confluent Points
- Yuan Source point for involved organ in chronic illness
- He Sea point can also be used for chronic illness
- Xi-Cleft point for acute illness

- Jingwell points in emergency conditions – such as convulsions, collapse, or coma

9. Points with Specific Effects – eg ST38 for frozen shoulder

10. New Points – eg Tim-Mee point in smoking addiction

11. Micro-Acupuncture Systems:

    - Ear
    - Hand
    - Foot
    - Scalp

Try to determine the patient's reactivity status – are they likely to be a Strong Responder or Hyper Reactor?

This will give you a list of possible points for the day's treatment.

Final Prescription

Now come up with the final prescription for which points you will use today.

Practical Tips

Remember to keep your points to the minimum necessary.

As a rule of thumb at the First Treatment avoid local points – use 1 or 2 well-chosen distal points or ear points. This reduces the risk of significantly aggravating Strong Responders and Hyper Reactors.

In general treat:

- Hyper Acute Conditions daily until settled – eg Acute Locked Back
- Acute Conditions in general treat every 2 –3 days until

settled

- With Hyper Acute and Acute Conditions, it may be worthwhile having a "booster treatment" about 1 week after the condition settles

- Chronic Conditions treat every 1 to 4 weeks

Anton Jayasuriya used to say that a chimpanzee can be trained to do acupuncture and can help 50% of people, a good acupuncturist can help 70% of people, a master acupuncturist can help 80% – and anyone who can help 100% is a fool or a liar!

Geoff Greenbaum considered that the art of acupuncture was the treatment of reactive points on the body surface and knowing which of these reactive points to treat on a given day.

He saw the prime effect of acupuncture as homoeostatic.

It is wisely said that the master acupuncturist uses 1 point only.

Needling can be superficial or deep, gentle or strong – as long as DeQi is elicited.

Felix Mann used to specialise in treating the patient very gently with just 1 needle.

Special point combinations

Influential Points

- BL11 – bone, cartilage, joints

- GB34 / LR3 – muscles, tendons

- LU9 – blood vessels, circulatory system

- CV17 – respiratory system, Qi

- CV12 – hollow organs, Fu

- LR13 – solid organs, Zang

- BL17 – blood
- GB39 - marrow

Area Of Influence Points

- LI4 - face
- LU7 – side of neck
- PC6 – chest & epigastrium
- ST36 – abdomen
- SP6 – pelvis & pelvic organs & inner legs
- BL40 – back & back of legs

Command Points

- GV26 – collapse, resuscitation
- LI4 – face & mouth
- LU7 – head, back, neck
- ST36 - abdomen
- BL40 - back

Alarm and Associated Points – Back Shu and Mu Front Points

For disorders of specific organs

- Lung – Mu Front Point LU1, Back Shu Point BL13
- Large Intestine – ST25, BL25
- Stomach – CV12, BL21
- Spleen – LR13, BL20
- Heart – CV14, BL15

- Small Intestine – CV4, BL27
- Bladder – CV3, BL28
- Kidney – GB25, BL23
- Pericardium – CV17, BL14
- Triple Energiser – CV5, BL22
- Gallbladder – GB24, BL19
- Liver – LR14, BL18

Confluent Points

- SI3 + BL62 – Back, all spine, especially neck
- LU7 + KI6 – Anterior body, throat, chest, lung
- TE5 + GB41 – Lateral side of body
- PC6 + SP4 – Internal organs, especially gynaecological, heart, stomach, chest

Great Points

- LI4, ST36, SP6 (Felix Mann would add LR3 to this list as his favourite point)

Physiological Points – points with recognised physiological effects:

- Analgesic - LI4, ST44
- Anti-inflammatory - GV14, LI4, LI11, ST36, SP6
- Immune Enhancing - GV14, LI4, LI11, ST36, SP6
  - Anti-allergy - SP10
  - Tranquillising - GV15, GV20, LI4, PC6, HT7, (HT3)

- Tonifying for low vitality - GV14, LI4, ST36, SP6, (CV6)
- Homoeostatic – LI4, LI11, ST36, SP6

Periosteal Points – bony tender points as per Felix Mann:

- CTP's – cervical transverse processes
- Coracoid Process
- Lateral Epicondyle of elbow
- SIJ – sacroiliac joint
- ASIS – anterior superior iliac spine
- "SP9" – just above true SP9 on the medial condyle of the tibia
- "BL62" – 1 cun below the lateral malleolus of the ankle

Points with Specific Effects – such as:

- ST38 for frozen shoulder
- Tim-Mee point for smoking addiction
- Spheno-Palatine Ganglion for hayfever

REFERENCES

- Armati, Patricia and Chow, Roberta. "Pain – The person, the science, the clinical interface" IP Communications. Melbourne. 2015.

- Becker, Robert. "The Body Electric". 1985.

- Bianco G. "Fascial neuromodulation: an emerging concept linking acupuncture, fasciology, osteopathy and neuroscience." Eur J Transl Myol. 2019 Aug 27;29(3):8331. doi: 10.4081/ejtm.2019.8331. PMID: 31579478; PMCID: PMC6767840.

- Bischko, Johannes. "An Introduction To Acupuncture". 1985. Haug Publishers. Germany.

- Bischko, Johannes. "Intermediate Acupuncture – Volume II: Textbook". 1986. Haug Publishers. Germany.

- Chow, Roberta et al. "Efficacy of low-level laser therapy in the management of neck pain: a systematic review and meta-analysis of randomised placebo or active-treatment controlled trials". Lancet 2009 Dec 5; 374(9705):1897-908.

- Chow, Roberta. "Dose Dilemmas in Low Level Laser Therapy – The Effects of Different Paradigms and Historical Perspectives". Laser Therapy. 2001;13:102-109.

- Chow, Roberta. Presentation on laser acupuncture at ICMART, Gold Coast, Australia. October 2019.

- Dorsher PT in "Myofascial Trigger Points – Comprehensive

diagnosis and treatment" edited by Irnich, Dominik. Churchill Livingstone Elsevier. 2009.

- Dorsher PT, Chiang P. "Neuroembryology of the Acupuncture Principal Meridians: Part 3. The Head and Neck". Med Acupunct. 2018 Apr 1; 30 (2):80-88
- Dorsher PT. "Can classical acupuncture points and trigger points be compared in the treatment of pain disorders? Birch's analysis revisited". J Altern Complement Med. 2008 May; 14(4):353-9.
- Dorsher PT. "Myofascial referred-pain data provide physiologic evidence of acupuncture meridians". J Pain. 2009 Jul; 10(7):723-31. Epub 2009 May 05.
- Filshie, Jacqueline; White, Adrian; Cummings, Mike. "Medical Acupuncture – A Western Scientific Approach". 2nd Edition. Elsevier. 2016.
- Finando, Steven; Finando, Donna. "Qi, Acupuncture, and the Fascia: A Reconsideration of the Fundamental Principles of Acupuncture". The Journal Of Alternative And Complementary Medicine, Volume 18, Number 9, 2012, pp. 880–886.
- Gerber, Richard. "Vibrational Medicine". Third Edition 2001. Bear & Company. Rochester, Vermont.
- Greenbaum, Geoff. Presentation on "15 Year Prospective Trial of Acupuncture in a Hospital Out-Patient Clinic with 1058 patients" at ICMART. 2002.
- Hamblin, Michael R. "Handbook of Photomedicine." 2013. CRC Press. USA. "Low Level Laser Therapy in the Treatment of Pain" Dr. Roberta Chow pp. 591-601.
- Hamblin, Michael R. "Shining light on the head: Photobiomodulation for brain disorders". BBA Clin. 2016 Dec; 6: 113–124. Elsevier.

- Hamblin, Michael R. et al. "Low-Level Light Therapy: Photobiomodulation". Bellingham, Washington, USA: SPIE Press, 2018. Series: Tutorial texts in optical engineering; volume TT115. Chapter 17 "LLLT Treatment of Pain: Clinical Applications" pp. 255-286 by Roberta Chow.
- Hoon Chung, Tianhong Dai, Sulbha K Sharma, Ying-Ying Huang, James D Carroll, Michael R Hamblin. "The nuts and bolts of low-level laser (light) therapy". Ann Biomed Eng. 2012 Feb;40(2):516-33.
- Hunt, Valerie and Massey, Wayne. "A Study of Structural Neuromuscular, Energy Field and Emotional Approaches". 1977. UCLA.
- Jayasuriya, Anton. "Clinical Acupuncture". B. Jain. India.
- Kilner, Walter. "The Human Aura". 1965. New York.
- Kim, Bong-Han. "Developmental and Comparative Biological Study of Primo Vascular System". Journal of Acupuncture and Meridian Studies. 5 (5): 248–255. doi:10.1016/j.jams.2012.07.016
- Mann, Felix. "Reinventing Acupuncture". 2nd edition. Free download at https://kupdf.net/download/felix-mann-reinventing-acupuncture-a-new-concepbookfiorg_59df20d308bbc5db0ee65861_pdf
- Motoyama, Hiyoshi. " The Functional Relationship Between Yoga Asanas and Acupuncture Meridians." 1979.
- Nakamura, K, and Hiramatsu, M. "Ultra-weak photon emission from human hand: influence of temperature and oxygen concentration on emission." J Photochem Photobiol B. 2005 Aug 1;80(2):156-60. http://www.ncbi.nlm.nih.gov/pubmed/15935689
- Olms, J.S. "How To Stop Smoking: Effective New Acupuncture Point Discovered". America Journal of Acupuncture. Vol 9. No

3. July-September 1981. pp 257-260.

- Qigong practitioners shrinking a bladder tumour at a Chinese hospital can be seen at https://youtu.be/31rf74-DQfA

- Reich, Wilhelm. "The Discovery of the Orgone". 1942.

- Schneideman, Ian. "Medical Acupuncture – Acupuncture and the Inner Healer". 1988. Self-published.

- Shem, Samuel. "The House Of God". First Edition 1979. Random House.

- Soulie de Morant, George. "L'Acupuncture Chinoise". 1955. English edition "Chinese Acupuncture". Paradigm Publications. USA. 1994.

- Vickers, A. J., Cronin, A. M., Maschino, A. C., Lewith, G., MacPherson, H., Foster, N. E., et al. "Acupuncture for chronic pain: individual patient data meta-analysis." 2012. Arch. Intern. Med. 172, 1444–1453. doi: 10.1001/archinternmed.2012.3654.

- Vickers, A. J., Vertosick, E. A., Lewith, G., MacPherson, H., Foster, N. E., Sherman, K. J., et al. "Acupuncture for chronic pain: update of an individual patient data meta-analysis." 2017. J. Pain 19, 455–474. doi: 10.1016/j.jpain.2017.11.005.

- White, Adrian; Cummings, Mike; Filshie, Jacqueline. "An Introduction To Western Medical Acupuncture". 2nd Edition. Elsevier. 2018.

- Zhou W, Benharash P. "Effects and mechanisms of acupuncture based on the principle of meridians". J Acupunct Meridian Stud. 2014 Aug;7(4):190-3. doi: 10.1016/j.jams.2014.02.007. Epub 2014 Jun 24. PMID: 25151452.

Useful Books For TCM

Some of these books are out of print, but well worth reading if you can get a copy:

- "Ling Shu" – various translations including "Ling Shu or The Spiritual Pivot" translated by Wu Jing-Nuan. University of Hawaii Press. 1993.
- Hammer, Leon. "Dragon Rises, Red Bird Flies – Psychology and Chinese Medicine". Revised edition 2005. Eastland Press. USA
- Jayasuriya, Anton. "Clinical Acupuncture". B. Jain. India.
- Mann, Felix. "Textbook Of Acupuncture". 1987. Omnibus.

Made in the USA
Monee, IL
04 November 2026

67384022R00115